KIDNEY DISEASE DIET COOKBOOK FOR STAGE 3

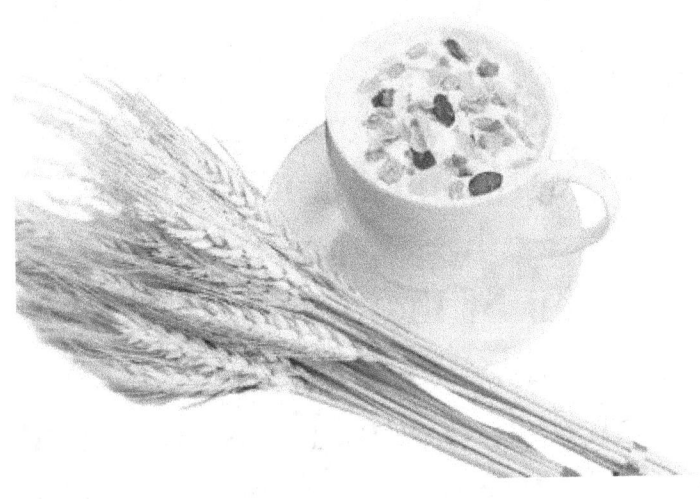

Delicious and Easy to make Low Sodium, Potassium and Phosphorus Recipes with 28-day Meal plan to manage CKD for Healthy Living

LAURA B. COLLINS

Copyright Laura B. Collins 2024

All rights reserved. No part of this publication may be reproduced, distributed, or transmitted in any form or by any means, including photocopying, recording, or other electronic or mechanical methods, without the prior written permission of the publisher, except in the case of brief quotations embodied in critical reviews and certain other noncommercial uses permitted by copyright law.

TABLE OF CONTENT

Chapter 1: Introduction to Kidney Disease and Stage 3 Diet 7
    Understanding Kidney Disease 7
    Overview of Stage 3 Chronic Kidney Disease (CKD) 9
    Importance of Diet in Managing Kidney Disease . 12

Chapter 2: Kidney-Friendly Eating Guidelines 15
    Nutritional Needs for Stage 3 CKD 15
    Key Nutrients to Monitor (Sodium, Potassium, Phosphorus) 17
    Tips for Meal Planning and Portion Control 20

Chapter 3: Breakfast Recipes 24
    Recipe 1: Vegetable Omelette 24
    Recipe 2: Greek Yogurt Parfait 25
    Recipe 3: Spinach and Feta Breakfast Wrap 26
    Recipe 4: Quinoa Breakfast Bowl 27
    Recipe 5: Avocado Toast with Poached Egg 28
    Recipe 6: Berry Chia Seed Pudding 30
    Recipe 7: Cottage Cheese Pancakes 31
    Recipe 8: Sweet Potato Breakfast Hash 32
    Recipe 9: Turkey and Vegetable Breakfast Skillet 33
    Recipe 10: Banana Nut Overnight Oats 35

Chapter 4: Lunch Recipes 37
    Recipe 1: Grilled Lemon Herb Chicken 37

Recipe 2: Quinoa Salad with Chickpeas and Vegetables 38

Recipe 3: Salmon and Asparagus Foil Packets 39

Recipe 4: Turkey and Vegetable Stir-Fry 41

Recipe 5: Lentil and Vegetable Soup 42

Recipe 6: Tuna Salad Lettuce Wraps 44

Recipe 7: Eggplant and Tomato Stacks 45

Recipe 8: Chicken and Vegetable Stir-Fry 46

Recipe 9: Black Bean and Corn Salad 48

Recipe 10: Turkey and Spinach Wrap 49

Chapter 5: Dinner Recipes 51

Recipe 1: Baked Lemon Herb Tilapia 51

Recipe 2: Vegetable Stir-Fried Brown Rice 52

Recipe 3: Turkey and Vegetable Skillet 54

Recipe 4: Lemon Garlic Shrimp Skewers 55

Recipe 5: Baked Chicken and Vegetable Casserole 56

Recipe 6: Quinoa Stuffed Bell Peppers 58

Recipe 7: Turkey Meatball and Vegetable Soup 60

Recipe 8: Baked Lemon Herb Chicken 61

Recipe 9: Vegetable and Tofu Stir-Fry 62

Recipe 10: Spaghetti Squash with Marinara Sauce 64

Chapter 6: Snack and Appetizers Recipes 65

Recipe 1: Cucumber and Cottage Cheese Bites 65

Recipe 2: Hummus and Veggie Platter 66

Recipe 3: Greek Yogurt Parfait 67
Recipe 4: Rice Cake with Almond Butter and Banana Slices 68
Recipe 5: Caprese Skewers 69
Recipe 6: Egg Salad Lettuce Wraps 71
Recipe 7: Edamame Hummus 72
Recipe 8: Zucchini Fritters 73
Recipe 9: Stuffed Mini Bell Peppers 75
Recipe 10: Baked Eggplant Chips 76

Chapter 7: Soups and Salads 78
Recipe 1: Minestrone Soup 78
Recipe 2: Chicken and Vegetable Soup 79
Recipe 3: Mixed Greens Salad with Lemon Vinaigrette 81
Recipe 4: Tomato Basil Soup 82
Recipe 5: Spinach and Strawberry Salad 83
Recipe 6: Lentil and Vegetable Soup 85
Recipe 7: Quinoa and Black Bean Salad 86
Recipe 8: Butternut Squash Soup 88
Recipe 9: Chickpea and Avocado Salad 89
Recipe 10: Cucumber and Tomato Salad 90

Chapter 8: Desserts and Treats 92
Recipe 1: Baked Apples with Cinnamon 92
Recipe 2: Berry Parfait 93
Recipe 3: Chia Seed Pudding 94

Recipe 4: Frozen Banana Bites 95
Recipe 5: Vanilla Rice Pudding 97
Recipe 6: Coconut Yogurt Parfait 98
Recipe 7: No-Bake Energy Bites 99
Recipe 8: Peach Frozen Yogurt 100
Recipe 9: Chocolate Avocado Mousse 102
Recipe 10: Frozen Grape Skewers 103
Chapter 9: Herbal Tea Recipes for kidney support .. 105
Recipe 1: Dandelion Root Tea 105
Recipe 2: Nettle Leaf Tea 106
Recipe 3: Marshmallow Root Tea 106
Recipe 4: Corn Silk Tea 107
Recipe 5: Ginger Turmeric Tea 108
Chapter 10: Low-Sodium Infused water Recipes 110
Recipe 1: Cucumber Mint Infused Water 110
Recipe 2: Citrus Basil Infused Water 111
Recipe 3: Berry Rosemary Infused Water 112
Recipe 4: Pineapple Ginger Infused Water 113
Recipe 5: Watermelon Basil Infused Water 114
Chapter 11: 28-Day Meal plan 115
CONCLUSION 190

Chapter 1: Introduction to Kidney Disease and Stage 3 Diet

Understanding Kidney Disease

Kidney disease, also known as renal disease, is a condition that affects the kidneys' ability to function properly. These bean-shaped organs play a crucial role in maintaining overall health by filtering waste products and excess fluids from the blood, regulating blood pressure, and producing hormones that help control red blood cell production and electrolyte balance. When the kidneys are damaged or diseased, their ability to perform these vital functions becomes compromised, leading to a range of health issues.

Section 1: Anatomy and Function of the Kidneys

The kidneys are located on either side of the spine, just below the rib cage. Each kidney contains millions of tiny structures called nephrons, which are responsible for filtering waste and excess fluids from the blood. The nephrons consist of a glomerulus, a cluster of blood vessels where filtration occurs, and a tubule, which reabsorbs essential substances back into the bloodstream while excreting waste products as urine.

Section 2: Types and Stages of Kidney Disease

There are several types of kidney disease, each with its own causes, symptoms, and treatment options. Chronic kidney disease (CKD) is a progressive condition that develops slowly over time and can eventually lead to kidney failure if left untreated. Acute kidney injury (AKI), on the other hand, is a sudden and temporary loss of kidney function often caused by severe illness, injury, or medication toxicity.

CKD is categorized into five stages based on the level of kidney function, with stage 1 being the mildest and stage 5 indicating kidney failure. Early stages of CKD may be asymptomatic or present with mild symptoms such as fatigue, swelling, and changes in urination patterns. As the disease progresses, symptoms may worsen and complications such as high blood pressure, anemia, and bone disease may develop.

Section 3: Causes and Risk Factors

Kidney disease can be caused by a variety of factors, including:

Diabetes: High blood sugar levels can damage the blood vessels in the kidneys over time, leading to kidney damage.

High blood pressure: Hypertension can strain the blood vessels in the kidneys, causing them to become damaged and reducing their ability to filter waste.

Other medical conditions: Conditions such as autoimmune diseases, polycystic kidney disease, and urinary tract infections can also contribute to kidney damage.

Lifestyle factors: Smoking, obesity, poor diet, and lack of exercise can increase the risk of developing kidney disease.

Medications and toxins: Certain medications, as well as exposure to environmental toxins such as heavy metals, can damage the kidneys.

Overview of Stage 3 Chronic Kidney Disease (CKD)

Chronic kidney disease (CKD) is a progressive condition characterized by the gradual loss of kidney function over time. Stage 3 CKD is a critical juncture in the progression of the disease, as it represents a moderate decrease in kidney function and requires close monitoring and management to prevent further decline.

Section 1: Understanding Stage 3 CKD

In Stage 3 CKD, the kidneys are still able to perform their essential functions, but their ability to filter waste products and excess fluids from the blood is significantly reduced. This can lead to an accumulation of toxins in the body, as well as imbalances in electrolytes and fluid levels. While some individuals with Stage 3 CKD may experience few or no symptoms, others may begin to notice signs of kidney dysfunction, such as fatigue, swelling, changes in urination patterns, and elevated blood pressure.

Section 2: Diagnostic Criteria and Testing

Diagnosing Stage 3 CKD typically involves a combination of blood tests, urine tests, and imaging studies to assess kidney function and determine the underlying cause of the disease. Common tests used to diagnose CKD include:

Serum creatinine test: Measures the level of creatinine, a waste product produced by muscle metabolism, in the blood. Elevated creatinine levels may indicate reduced kidney function.

Estimated glomerular filtration rate (eGFR): Estimates the rate at which the kidneys filter waste from the blood. A lower eGFR value indicates decreased kidney function.

Urinalysis: Examines a sample of urine for the presence of protein, blood, or other abnormalities that may indicate kidney damage.

Imaging studies: such as ultrasound, CT scan, or MRI may be used to evaluate the size and structure of the kidneys and identify any abnormalities.

Section 3: Treatment and Management

The goal of treatment for Stage 3 CKD is to slow the progression of the disease, manage symptoms, and reduce the risk of complications. This typically involves a combination of lifestyle modifications, medications, and medical interventions. Key components of treatment may include:

Dietary changes: Adopting a kidney-friendly diet that is low in sodium, phosphorus, and potassium can help reduce the workload on the kidneys and prevent further damage.

Blood pressure management: Controlling high blood pressure is crucial for preserving kidney function and reducing the risk of cardiovascular complications. This may involve lifestyle changes, such as regular exercise and stress management, as well as medications.

Medications: Certain medications, such as angiotensin-converting enzyme (ACE) inhibitors or angiotensin II receptor blockers (ARBs), may be prescribed to help lower blood pressure and protect kidney function.

Monitoring and follow-up care: Regular monitoring of kidney function, blood pressure, and other health markers is essential for managing Stage 3 CKD effectively. Close communication with healthcare providers and adherence to treatment recommendations can help prevent complications and improve outcomes.

Importance of Diet in Managing Kidney Disease

Diet plays a crucial role in the management of kidney disease, especially in Stage 3 Chronic Kidney Disease (CKD). A kidney-friendly diet can help slow the progression of the disease, manage symptoms, and reduce the risk of complications. In this chapter, we will explore the importance of diet in managing kidney disease and discuss key dietary principles for individuals with Stage 3 CKD.

Section 1: Managing Fluid and Electrolyte Balance

One of the primary functions of the kidneys is to regulate fluid and electrolyte balance in the body. In Stage 3 CKD, the kidneys may have difficulty excreting excess fluid and electrolytes, leading to fluid retention, electrolyte imbalances, and hypertension. A kidney-friendly diet focuses on:

Limiting sodium intake: Excessive sodium consumption can contribute to fluid retention and high blood pressure. Individuals with Stage 3 CKD are typically advised to limit their sodium intake to <2,000 mg per day.

Monitoring potassium and phosphorus: Elevated levels of potassium and phosphorus in the blood can be harmful to individuals with CKD. Foods high in potassium and phosphorus, such as bananas, oranges, tomatoes, dairy products, and processed foods, should be limited or avoided.

Maintaining adequate fluid intake: While fluid restriction may be necessary in later stages of CKD, individuals with Stage 3 CKD are generally encouraged to drink enough fluids to stay hydrated, unless otherwise advised by their healthcare provider.

Section 2: Protein Intake and Kidney Function

Protein is an essential nutrient for overall health, but excessive protein intake can put strain on the kidneys and may accelerate the progression of kidney disease. In Stage 3 CKD, individuals are often advised to:

Monitor protein intake: Aim for a moderate protein intake of 0.6-0.8 grams of protein per kilogram of body weight per day. This can help reduce the workload on the kidneys while still providing adequate nutrition.

Choose high-quality protein sources: Opt for lean protein sources such as poultry, fish, eggs, and plant-based proteins like beans, lentils, and tofu. These sources are lower in phosphorus and potassium compared to red meat and processed meats.

Section 3: Meeting Nutritional Needs

Individuals with Stage 3 CKD may be at risk for malnutrition due to dietary restrictions, reduced appetite, and impaired nutrient absorption. It's important to:

Focus on nutrient-dense foods: Choose foods that are rich in essential nutrients such as vitamins, minerals, and antioxidants. This includes fruits, vegetables, whole grains, and lean proteins.

Consider vitamin and mineral supplementation: In some cases, individuals with CKD may require supplementation with certain vitamins and minerals, such as vitamin D, iron, and B vitamins. Consultation with a healthcare provider or registered dietitian is recommended to determine individualized supplement needs.

Chapter 2: Kidney-Friendly Eating Guidelines

Nutritional Needs for Stage 3 CKD

Stage 3 Chronic Kidney Disease (CKD) represents a critical phase in the progression of kidney disease, where the kidneys may still be functioning, but their ability to filter waste products and maintain fluid and electrolyte balance is significantly impaired. In this chapter, we will delve into the specific nutritional needs of individuals with Stage 3 CKD and discuss dietary strategies to support kidney health.

Section 1: Protein Intake

Protein is an essential nutrient that plays a crucial role in maintaining muscle mass, supporting immune function, and repairing tissues. However, in Stage 3 CKD, excessive protein intake can put strain on the kidneys and may accelerate the progression of kidney disease. To meet nutritional needs while minimizing kidney workload, individuals with Stage 3 CKD are advised to:

Opt for high-quality protein sources: Choose lean protein sources such as poultry, fish, eggs, and plant-based proteins like beans, lentils, and tofu. These sources are lower in phosphorus and potassium compared to red meat and processed meats.

Monitor protein intake: Aim for a moderate protein intake of 0.6-0.8 grams of protein per kilogram of body weight per day. This can help reduce the workload on the kidneys while still providing adequate nutrition.

Section 2: Fluid Management

Maintaining fluid balance is essential for individuals with Stage 3 CKD, as impaired kidney function can lead to fluid retention and electrolyte imbalances. To manage fluid intake effectively, individuals are encouraged to:

Monitor fluid intake: Keep track of fluid intake throughout the day and avoid excessive consumption of fluids, especially those high in sodium and sugar.

Choose hydrating beverages: Opt for water, herbal teas, and diluted fruit juices as primary sources of hydration, and limit intake of caffeinated and alcoholic beverages, which can contribute to dehydration.

Section 3: Electrolyte Balance

Electrolytes such as sodium, potassium, and phosphorus play a crucial role in maintaining cellular function and fluid balance in the body. In Stage 3 CKD, electrolyte imbalances can occur due to impaired kidney function. To manage electrolyte balance effectively, individuals are advised to:

Limit sodium intake: Reduce consumption of processed and packaged foods, which are typically high in sodium. Choose fresh, whole foods and use herbs, spices, and lemon juice to add flavor to meals.

Monitor potassium and phosphorus intake: Limit intake of potassium and phosphorus-rich foods such as bananas, oranges, tomatoes, dairy products, and processed foods. Opt for low-potassium and low-phosphorus alternatives whenever possible.

Key Nutrients to Monitor (Sodium, Potassium, Phosphorus)

In Stage 3 Chronic Kidney Disease (CKD), managing the intake of certain nutrients becomes crucial to prevent complications and slow the progression of kidney disease. Sodium, potassium, and phosphorus are three key nutrients that require close monitoring, as imbalances can exacerbate kidney dysfunction and contribute to adverse health outcomes. In this chapter, we will explore the importance of monitoring sodium, potassium, and phosphorus intake and provide practical strategies for maintaining optimal levels of these nutrients.

Section 1: Sodium

Sodium is an essential mineral that plays a critical role in maintaining fluid balance, nerve function, and muscle contractions in the body. However, excessive sodium intake can lead to fluid retention, high blood pressure, and cardiovascular complications, particularly in individuals with kidney disease. To manage sodium intake effectively, individuals with Stage 3 CKD are advised to:

Limit processed and packaged foods: Processed and packaged foods are often high in sodium, so it's essential to read food labels carefully and choose low-sodium or sodium-free alternatives whenever possible.

Use herbs and spices: Instead of relying on salt to flavor meals, experiment with herbs, spices, lemon juice, vinegar, and other flavor-enhancing ingredients to add taste to dishes without increasing sodium intake.

Be mindful of condiments and sauces: Many condiments and sauces, such as ketchup, soy sauce, barbecue sauce, and salad dressings, are high in sodium. Opt for low-sodium or homemade versions, or use them sparingly.

Section 2: Potassium

Potassium is a mineral that helps regulate fluid balance, nerve function, and muscle contractions in the body. While potassium is essential for overall health, individuals with Stage 3 CKD may need to limit their intake to prevent hyperkalemia (elevated potassium levels), which can be harmful to the heart and other organs. To manage potassium intake effectively, individuals are advised to:

Choose low-potassium foods: Limit consumption of potassium-rich foods such as bananas, oranges, tomatoes, potatoes, and dairy products. Instead, opt for low-potassium alternatives such as apples, berries, cabbage, and green beans.

Practice portion control: Even low-potassium foods can contribute to elevated potassium levels if consumed in large quantities. Be mindful of portion sizes and spread potassium-rich foods throughout the day to avoid overloading the kidneys.

Section 3: Phosphorus

Phosphorus is a mineral that plays a crucial role in bone health, energy metabolism, and cell function. However, individuals with Stage 3 CKD may need to limit their phosphorus intake to prevent hyperphosphatemia (elevated phosphorus levels), which can contribute to bone disease, cardiovascular complications, and other health issues. To manage phosphorus intake effectively, individuals are advised to:

Limit phosphorus-rich foods: Reduce consumption of phosphorus-rich foods such as dairy products, nuts, seeds, whole grains, and processed foods containing phosphate additives.

Choose phosphorus binders: In some cases, individuals with Stage 3 CKD may be prescribed phosphorus binders, medications that help prevent the absorption of phosphorus from food. These medications should be taken as directed by a healthcare provider.

By monitoring sodium, potassium, and phosphorus intake and making dietary adjustments as needed, individuals with Stage 3 CKD can help support kidney health and reduce the risk of complications associated with kidney disease.

Tips for Meal Planning and Portion Control

Meal planning and portion control are essential components of managing Stage 3 Chronic Kidney Disease (CKD) effectively. By carefully selecting nutritious foods and controlling portion sizes, individuals can better manage their nutrient intake and support kidney health. In this chapter, we will explore practical tips and strategies for meal planning and portion control for individuals with Stage 3 CKD.

Section 1: Plan Ahead

Create a weekly meal plan: Take some time at the beginning of each week to plan out your meals and snacks. This can help ensure that you have nutritious options available and reduce the temptation to make unhealthy choices on the fly.

Make a shopping list: Based on your meal plan, create a shopping list of ingredients you'll need for the week. Stick to your list while shopping to avoid impulse purchases of foods that may not be kidney-friendly.

Batch cook and meal prep: Consider preparing larger batches of meals and portioning them out into individual servings to have on hand throughout the week. This can save time and make it easier to stick to your meal plan.

Section 2: Choose Kidney-Friendly Foods

Focus on whole foods: Choose whole, unprocessed foods whenever possible, such as fruits, vegetables, lean proteins, and whole grains. These foods are generally lower in sodium, potassium, and phosphorus and higher in essential nutrients compared to processed options.

Read food labels: Pay attention to food labels and nutrition facts to identify foods that are high in sodium, potassium, or phosphorus. Look for low-sodium, low-potassium, and low-phosphorus options, and aim to choose foods with less than 20% of the daily value for these nutrients per serving.

Incorporate variety: Include a variety of foods from all food groups in your meals and snacks to ensure that you're getting a wide range of nutrients. Experiment with different flavors, textures, and cooking methods to keep meals interesting and enjoyable.

Section 3: Practice Portion Control

Use smaller plates: Opt for smaller plates and bowls to help control portion sizes and prevent overeating. This can help trick your brain into thinking you're eating more than you actually are.

Measure portions: Use measuring cups, spoons, and kitchen scales to portion out foods and ingredients accurately. This can help prevent portion distortion and ensure that you're consuming appropriate serving sizes.

Fill half your plate with vegetables: Vegetables are low in calories and high in nutrients, making them an excellent choice for filling up your plate without going overboard on calories or nutrients that may be harmful to kidney health.

Section 4: Listen to Your Body

Practice mindful eating: Pay attention to hunger and fullness cues and eat slowly and mindfully. Stop eating when you feel satisfied, rather than waiting until you're overly full.

Stay hydrated: Drink plenty of fluids throughout the day, as dehydration can sometimes be mistaken for hunger. Aim to drink at least 8-10 cups of water per day, unless otherwise advised by your healthcare provider.

Seek support: Consider working with a registered dietitian or nutritionist who specializes in kidney health to develop a personalized meal plan that meets your individual needs and preferences.

Chapter 3: Breakfast Recipes

Recipe 1: Vegetable Omelette

Prep Time: 10 minutes

Serving Size: 1 omelette

Ingredients:

2 eggs, 1/4 cup diced bell peppers

1/4 cup diced onions, 1/4 cup diced tomatoes

1 tablespoon chopped parsley, Salt and pepper to taste

Instructions:

In a bowl, whisk together the eggs with salt and pepper.

Heat a non-stick skillet over medium heat and lightly coat with cooking spray.

Pour the egg mixture into the skillet and swirl to evenly distribute.

Cook for 2-3 minutes until the edges start to set.

Sprinkle the diced vegetables and parsley evenly over one half of the omelette.

Gently fold the other half of the omelette over the vegetables.

Cook for an additional 2-3 minutes until the omelette is cooked through.

Nutritional Facts (per serving):

Calories: 180

Protein: 14g

Carbohydrates: 5g

Tips:

Use fresh herbs like basil or thyme for added flavor without extra sodium.

Recipe 2: Greek Yogurt Parfait

Prep Time: 5 minutes

Serving Size: 1 parfait

Ingredients:

1/2 cup plain Greek yogurt, 1/4 cup sliced strawberries

1/4 cup blueberries, 1 tablespoon chopped walnuts

Instructions:

In a glass or bowl, layer the Greek yogurt with sliced strawberries and blueberries.

Sprinkle chopped walnuts on top for added crunch.

Drizzle with honey if desired.

Nutritional Facts (per serving):

Calories: 180

Protein: 15g

Carbohydrates: 15g

Tips:

Opt for plain Greek yogurt to avoid added sugars and artificial flavors.

Recipe 3: Spinach and Feta Breakfast Wrap

Prep Time: 10 minutes

Serving Size: 1 wrap

Ingredients:

1 whole grain tortilla, 2 eggs, scrambled

1/4 cup fresh spinach leaves, 2 tablespoons crumbled feta cheese, Salt and pepper to taste.

Instructions:

Warm the tortilla in a skillet over medium heat.

In the same skillet, scramble the eggs until cooked through.

Lay the warm tortilla flat and top with fresh spinach leaves.

Spoon the scrambled eggs onto the spinach.

Sprinkle with crumbled feta cheese.

Season with salt and pepper to taste.

Fold the sides of the tortilla over the filling and roll it up into a wrap.

Nutritional Facts (per serving):

Calories: 280

Protein: 17g

Carbohydrates: 20g

Tips:

Choose a whole grain tortilla for added fiber and nutrients.

Recipe 4: Quinoa Breakfast Bowl

Prep Time: 15 minutes

Serving Size: 1 bowl

Ingredients:

1/2 cup cooked quinoa, 1/4 cup sliced strawberries

1/4 cup blueberries, 2 tablespoons chopped almonds

Instructions:

In a bowl, layer cooked quinoa with sliced strawberries and blueberries.

Top with chopped almonds for added crunch.

Drizzle with honey if desired.

Serve warm or cold as a nutritious and filling breakfast option.

Nutritional Facts (per serving):

Carbohydrates: 42g

Fiber: 6g

Sodium: 10mg

Tips:

Cook quinoa in low-sodium vegetable or chicken broth for added flavor.

Recipe 5: Avocado Toast with Poached Egg

Prep Time: 15 minutes

Serving Size: 1 toast

Ingredients:

1 slice of whole grain bread, toasted, 1/2 ripe avocado, mashed, 1 large egg, Salt and pepper to taste.

Instructions:

Toast the slice of whole grain bread until golden brown.

While the bread is toasting, bring a small pot of water to a simmer.

Crack the egg into a small bowl or ramekin.

Carefully slide the egg into the simmering water and poach for 3-4 minutes until the whites are set but the yolk is still runny.

Remove the poached egg from the water with a slotted spoon and drain on a paper towel.

Spread the mashed avocado evenly onto the toasted bread.

Place the poached egg on top of the avocado.

Nutritional Facts (per serving):

Carbohydrates: 18g

Fiber: 6g

Sodium: 180mg

Tips:

Add a sprinkle of red pepper flakes or a squeeze of lemon juice for extra flavor.

Recipe 6: Berry Chia Seed Pudding

Prep Time: 5 minutes (plus chilling time)

Serving Size: 1 pudding

Ingredients:

2 tablespoons chia seeds, 1/2 cup unsweetened almond milk

1/4 cup mixed berries (such as strawberries, blueberries, and raspberries).

Instructions:

In a small bowl or jar, mix together chia seeds and almond milk.

Stir well to combine, then cover and refrigerate for at least 2 hours or overnight until thickened.

Once the chia pudding has set, layer it with mixed berries in a serving glass or bowl.

Serve chilled as a nutritious and satisfying breakfast or snack.

Nutritional Facts (per serving):

Protein: 4g

Fiber: 9g

Sodium: 60mg

Tips:

Experiment with different types of milk, such as coconut milk or soy milk, for variety.

Recipe 7: Cottage Cheese Pancakes

Prep Time: 10 minutes

Serving Size: 2 pancakes

Ingredients:

1/2 cup low-fat cottage cheese, 2 eggs, 2 tablespoons almond flour

1/2 teaspoon vanilla extract, Cooking spray or oil for frying.

Instructions:

In a blender or food processor, combine cottage cheese, eggs, almond flour, and vanilla extract.

Blend until smooth and well combined.

Heat a non-stick skillet or griddle over medium heat and lightly coat with cooking spray or oil.

Pour small portions of the batter onto the skillet to form pancakes.

Cook for 2-3 minutes on each side until golden brown and cooked through.

Nutritional Facts (per serving):

Protein: 20g

Fiber: 1g

Sodium: 360mg

Tips:

Adjust the consistency of the batter by adding more almond flour for thicker pancakes or more milk for thinner pancakes.

Recipe 8: Sweet Potato Breakfast Hash

Prep Time: 20 minutes

Serving Size: 1 cup

Ingredients:

1 small sweet potato, diced, 1/4 cup diced bell peppers

1/4 cup diced onions, 1/4 cup cooked black beans

1 teaspoon olive oil, Salt and pepper to taste.

Instructions:

Heat olive oil in a skillet over medium heat.

Add diced sweet potatoes and cook for 5-7 minutes until lightly browned and tender.

Add diced bell peppers and onions to the skillet and cook for an additional 3-4 minutes until vegetables are softened.

Stir in cooked black beans and season with salt and pepper to taste.

Cook for another 2-3 minutes until everything is heated through.

Nutritional Facts (per serving):

Protein: 5g

Fiber: 6g

Sodium: 160mg

Tips:

Top with a poached egg or avocado slices for added protein and flavor.

Sprinkle with chopped fresh herbs like cilantro or parsley before serving.

Recipe 9: Turkey and Vegetable Breakfast Skillet

Prep Time: 15 minutes

Serving Size: 1 cup

Ingredients:

2 ounces lean turkey sausage, sliced, 1/4 cup diced bell peppers, 1/4 cup diced onions,

1/4 cup diced tomatoes, 1/4 cup baby spinach leaves, 2 eggs.

Instructions:

In a skillet, cook turkey sausage slices over medium heat until browned and cooked through.

Add diced bell peppers and onions to the skillet and cook for 3-4 minutes until softened.

Stir in diced tomatoes and baby spinach leaves, and cook until spinach wilts.

Make two wells in the skillet and crack an egg into each well.

Cook until the eggs are set to your desired level of doneness.

Nutritional Facts (per serving):

Protein: 20g

Fiber: 3g

Sodium: 390mg

Tips:

Serve with whole grain toast or a side of fruit for a complete meal.

Recipe 10: Banana Nut Overnight Oats

Prep Time: 5 minutes (plus chilling time)

Serving Size: 1 bowl

Ingredients:

1/2 cup old-fashioned oats, 1/2 cup unsweetened almond milk, 1/2 ripe banana, mashed,

1 tablespoon chopped walnuts, 1 teaspoon honey.

Instructions:

In a bowl or jar, combine old-fashioned oats, unsweetened almond milk, mashed banana, and chopped walnuts.

Stir well to combine, then cover and refrigerate overnight or for at least 4 hours until thickened.

Once the oats have absorbed the liquid and softened, stir again to mix everything evenly.

Drizzle with honey if desired for extra sweetness.

Nutritional Facts (per serving):

Protein: 8g

Fiber: 7g

Sodium: 80mg

Tips:

Add a sprinkle of cinnamon or a dash of vanilla extract for added flavor.

Chapter 4: Lunch Recipes

Recipe 1: Grilled Lemon Herb Chicken

Prep Time: 10 minutes

Cook Time: 15 minutes

Serving Size: 1 chicken breast

Ingredients:

1 boneless, skinless chicken breast, 1 tablespoon olive oil, 1 tablespoon lemon juice

1 teaspoon dried herbs (such as rosemary, thyme, or oregano), Salt and pepper to taste.

Instructions:

In a small bowl, whisk together olive oil, lemon juice, dried herbs, salt, and pepper.

Place the chicken breast in a shallow dish and pour the marinade over it.

Cover and refrigerate for at least 30 minutes to marinate.

Preheat grill or grill pan to medium-high heat.

Remove chicken breast from marinade and grill for 6-7 minutes on each side, or until cooked through.

Let it rest for a few minutes before slicing.

Serve with a side of steamed vegetables or a mixed green salad.

Nutritional Facts (per serving):

Protein: 25g

Fiber: 0g

Sodium: 80mg

Tips:

Use a meat thermometer to ensure the chicken reaches an internal temperature of 165°F (75°C).

Add minced garlic to the marinade for extra flavor.

Recipe 2: Quinoa Salad with Chickpeas and Vegetables

Prep Time: 15 minutes

Cook Time: 15 minutes

Serving Size: 1 cup

Ingredients:

1/2 cup cooked quinoa, 1/4 cup cooked chickpeas, 1/4 cup diced cucumber, 1/4 cup diced bell peppers

2 tablespoons chopped fresh parsley, 1 tablespoon lemon juice, 1 tablespoon olive oil, Salt and pepper to taste.

Instructions:

In a large bowl, combine cooked quinoa, chickpeas, cucumber, bell peppers, and parsley.

In a small bowl, whisk together lemon juice, olive oil, salt, and pepper.

Pour the dressing over the quinoa mixture and toss to coat evenly.

Serve chilled or at room temperature as a refreshing and nutritious salad option.

Nutritional Facts (per serving):

Protein: 8g

Fiber: 6g

Sodium: 100mg

Tips:

Add diced tomatoes or avocado for extra flavor and nutrients.

Recipe 3: Salmon and Asparagus Foil Packets

Prep Time: 10 minutes

Cook Time: 20 minutes

Serving Size: 1 foil packet

Ingredients:

1 salmon fillet, 1/2 cup asparagus spears, 1/4 cup cherry tomatoes, halved

1 tablespoon olive oil, 1 tablespoon lemon juice

1 teaspoon minced garlic, Salt and pepper to taste.

Instructions:

Preheat the oven to 375°F (190°C).

Place a salmon fillet on a piece of aluminum foil.

Arrange asparagus spears and cherry tomatoes around the salmon.

In a small bowl, whisk together olive oil, lemon juice, minced garlic, salt, and pepper.

Drizzle the mixture over the salmon and vegetables.

Fold the edges of the foil to create a sealed packet.

Place the foil packet on a baking sheet and bake for 15-20 minutes, or until the salmon is cooked through.

Nutritional Facts (per serving):

Protein: 25g

Fiber: 2g

Sodium: 100mg

Tips:

Customize with your favorite vegetables, such as bell peppers or zucchini.

Recipe 4: Turkey and Vegetable Stir-Fry

Prep Time: 15 minutes

Cook Time: 10 minutes

Serving Size: 1 cup

Ingredients:

4 ounces lean turkey breast, thinly sliced

1 cup mixed vegetables (such as bell peppers, snap peas, and carrots)

1 tablespoon low-sodium soy sauce, 1 teaspoon sesame oil, 1 teaspoon minced ginger

1 clove garlic, minced, 1 tablespoon chopped green onions.

Instructions:

Heat sesame oil in a large skillet or wok over medium-high heat.

Add minced ginger and garlic, and sauté for 1 minute until fragrant.

Add sliced turkey breast to the skillet and cook for 3-4 minutes until browned.

Add mixed vegetables to the skillet and stir-fry for an additional 3-4 minutes until tender-crisp.

Drizzle low-sodium soy sauce over the turkey and vegetables, and toss to combine.

Cook for another minute until heated through.

Sprinkle chopped green onions on top before serving.

Nutritional Facts (per serving):

Protein: 20g

Fat: 7g

Sodium: 300mg

Tips:

Add a splash of rice vinegar or lime juice for extra flavor.

Recipe 5: Lentil and Vegetable Soup

Prep Time: 10 minutes

Cook Time: 30 minutes

Serving Size: 1 cup

Ingredients:

1/2 cup dried green lentils, rinsed

4 cups low-sodium vegetable broth

1 carrot, diced, 1 celery stalk, diced, 1/2 onion, diced

1 garlic clove, minced, 1 teaspoon dried thyme.

Instructions:

In a large pot, combine dried lentils, vegetable broth, diced carrot, celery, onion, minced garlic, and dried thyme.

Bring the mixture to a boil over medium-high heat.

Reduce the heat to low, cover, and simmer for 25-30 minutes until the lentils and vegetables are tender.

Season with salt and pepper to taste.

Nutritional Facts (per serving):

Protein: 10g

Fiber: 10g

Sodium: 200mg

Tips:

Add leafy greens like spinach or kale during the last few minutes of cooking for extra nutrients.

Recipe 6: Tuna Salad Lettuce Wraps

Prep Time: 10 minutes

Serving Size: 2 lettuce wraps

Ingredients:

1 can (5 ounces) tuna in water, drained

2 tablespoons Greek yogurt, 1 tablespoon lemon juice, 1/4 cup diced celery

1/4 cup diced red onion, Salt and pepper to taste, 4 large lettuce leaves.

Instructions:

In a mixing bowl, combine tuna, Greek yogurt, lemon juice, diced celery, and diced red onion.

Mix well until all ingredients are evenly combined.

Season with salt and pepper to taste.

Spoon the tuna salad mixture onto lettuce leaves.

Wrap the lettuce leaves around the filling to form lettuce wraps.

Serve immediately as a light and protein-rich lunch option.

Nutritional Facts (per serving):

Protein: 15g

Fat: 5g

Sodium: 250mg

Tips:

Add chopped pickles or olives for extra flavor and texture.

Recipe 7: Eggplant and Tomato Stacks

Prep Time: 15 minutes

Cook Time: 20 minutes

Serving Size: 1 stack

Ingredients:

1 small eggplant, sliced into rounds, 2 tomatoes, sliced into rounds, 2 tablespoons olive oil

1 teaspoon dried Italian herbs, Salt and pepper to taste.

Instructions:

Preheat the oven to 375°F (190°C).

Place eggplant slices on a baking sheet lined with parchment paper.

Drizzle olive oil over the eggplant slices and sprinkle with dried Italian herbs, salt, and pepper.

Roast in the oven for 15-20 minutes until eggplant is tender.

Remove from the oven and let cool slightly.

Assemble stacks by layering eggplant slices with tomato slices.

Repeat layers until desired height is reached.

Serve warm as a flavorful and low-calorie lunch option.

Nutritional Facts (per serving):

Protein: 2g

Fat: 5g

Sodium: 10mg

Tips:

Top with fresh basil leaves or a sprinkle of grated Parmesan cheese before serving.

Drizzle with balsamic glaze for extra flavor.

Recipe 8: Chicken and Vegetable Stir-Fry

Prep Time: 15 minutes

Cook Time: 15 minutes

Serving Size: 1 cup

Ingredients:

4 ounces chicken breast, thinly sliced

1 cup mixed vegetables (such as broccoli, bell peppers, and snap peas)

2 tablespoons low-sodium soy sauce, 1 tablespoon olive oil, 1 teaspoon minced garlic, 1 teaspoon minced ginger.

Instructions:

Heat olive oil in a large skillet or wok over medium-high heat.

Add minced garlic and ginger, and sauté for 1 minute until fragrant.

Add sliced chicken breast to the skillet and cook for 3-4 minutes until browned.

Add mixed vegetables to the skillet and stir-fry for an additional 3-4 minutes until tender-crisp.

Drizzle low-sodium soy sauce over the chicken and vegetables, and toss to combine.

Cook for another minute until heated through.

Nutritional Facts (per serving):

Protein: 20g

Fat: 7g

Sodium: 300mg

Tips:

Add a splash of rice vinegar or lime juice for extra flavor.

Recipe 9: Black Bean and Corn Salad

Prep Time: 10 minutes

Serving Size: 1 cup

Ingredients:

1 can (15 ounces) black beans, drained and rinsed

1 cup frozen corn, thawed

1/2 cup diced red bell pepper, 1/4 cup chopped fresh cilantro, 2 tablespoons lime juice

1 tablespoon olive oil, 1 teaspoon ground cumin, Salt and pepper to taste.

Instructions:

In a large bowl, combine black beans, corn, diced red bell pepper, and chopped fresh cilantro.

In a small bowl, whisk together lime juice, olive oil, ground cumin, salt, and pepper.

Pour the dressing over the bean mixture and toss to coat evenly.

Serve chilled or at room temperature as a flavorful and protein-rich salad option.

Nutritional Facts (per serving):

Protein: 6g

Fat: 5g

Sodium: 200mg

Tips:

Add diced avocado or cherry tomatoes for extra flavor and nutrients.

Serve with baked tortilla chips or whole grain crackers for a satisfying crunch.

Recipe 10: Turkey and Spinach Wrap

Prep Time: 10 minutes

Serving Size: 1 wrap

Ingredients:

1 whole grain tortilla, 2 slices turkey breast, 1/4 cup hummus

1/2 cup fresh spinach leaves, 1/4 cup shredded carrots.

Instructions:

Lay the whole grain tortilla flat on a clean surface.

Spread hummus evenly over the tortilla.

Layer turkey breast slices, fresh spinach leaves, and shredded carrots on top of the hummus.

Roll the tortilla tightly into a wrap.

Slice in half if desired and serve immediately or wrap in foil for later.

Nutritional Facts (per serving):

Protein: 15g

Fat: 8g

Sodium: 350mg

Tips:

Add sliced cucumber or bell peppers for extra crunch and flavor.

Chapter 5: Dinner Recipes

Recipe 1: Baked Lemon Herb Tilapia

Prep Time: 10 minutes

Cook Time: 20 minutes

Serving Size: 1 fillet

Ingredients:

1 tilapia fillet, 1 tablespoon olive oil

1 tablespoon lemon juice

1 teaspoon dried herbs (such as thyme or dill), Salt and pepper to taste.

Instructions:

Preheat the oven to 375°F (190°C).

Place the tilapia fillet on a baking sheet lined with parchment paper.

Drizzle olive oil and lemon juice over the tilapia.

Sprinkle dried herbs, salt, and pepper evenly over the fillet.

Bake in the preheated oven for 15-20 minutes, or until the fish is cooked through and flakes easily with a fork.

Nutritional Facts (per serving):

Protein: 20g

Fat: 7g

Sodium: 70mg

Tips:

Garnish with fresh parsley or lemon slices before serving.

Recipe 2: Vegetable Stir-Fried Brown Rice

Prep Time: 10 minutes

Cook Time: 15 minutes

Serving Size: 1 cup

Ingredients:

1 cup cooked brown rice

1 cup mixed vegetables (such as bell peppers, broccoli, and carrots), 2 tablespoons low-sodium soy sauce

1 tablespoon olive oil, 1 teaspoon minced garlic, 1 teaspoon minced ginger.

Instructions:

Heat olive oil in a large skillet or wok over medium-high heat.

Add minced garlic and ginger, and sauté for 1 minute until fragrant.

Add mixed vegetables to the skillet and stir-fry for 3-4 minutes until tender-crisp.

Add cooked brown rice to the skillet and toss to combine with the vegetables.

Drizzle low-sodium soy sauce over the rice and vegetables, and stir-fry for another 2-3 minutes until heated through.

Nutritional Facts (per serving):

Protein: 5g

Fat: 5g

Sodium: 300mg

Tips:

Add cooked chicken breast or tofu for extra protein.

Sprinkle with sesame seeds or chopped green onions before serving.

Recipe 3: Turkey and Vegetable Skillet

Prep Time: 10 minutes

Cook Time: 20 minutes

Serving Size: 1 cup

Ingredients:

4 ounces lean ground turkey

1 cup mixed vegetables (such as bell peppers, zucchini, and mushrooms)

1 tablespoon olive oil, 1 teaspoon minced garlic

1 teaspoon dried Italian herbs, Salt and pepper to taste.

Instructions:

Heat olive oil in a large skillet over medium heat.

Add lean ground turkey to the skillet and cook until browned and cooked through.

Add mixed vegetables to the skillet and stir-fry for 5-7 minutes until tender.

Season with dried Italian herbs, salt, and pepper to taste.

Serve hot as a protein-rich and satisfying dinner option.

Nutritional Facts (per serving):

Protein: 20g

Fiber: 3g

Sodium: 250mg

Tips:

Serve over cooked quinoa or brown rice for a complete meal.

Recipe 4: Lemon Garlic Shrimp Skewers

Prep Time: 10 minutes

Cook Time: 5 minutes

Serving Size: 2 skewers

Ingredients:

8 large shrimp, peeled and deveined

1 tablespoon olive oil, 1 tablespoon lemon juice

1 teaspoon minced garlic, Salt and pepper to taste.

Instructions:

Preheat grill or grill pan to medium-high heat.

In a small bowl, whisk together olive oil, lemon juice, minced garlic, salt, and pepper.

Thread shrimp onto skewers and brush with the lemon garlic mixture.

Grill shrimp skewers for 2-3 minutes on each side, or until shrimp are pink and opaque.

Serve hot as a light and flavorful dinner option.

Nutritional Facts (per serving):

Protein: 20g

Fat: 4g

Sodium: 150mg

Tips:

Serve with grilled vegetables or a side salad for a balanced meal.

Use metal or soaked wooden skewers to prevent burning.

Recipe 5: Baked Chicken and Vegetable Casserole

Prep Time: 15 minutes

Cook Time: 30 minutes

Serving Size: 1 cup

Ingredients:

1 boneless, skinless chicken breast

1 cup mixed vegetables (such as broccoli, cauliflower, and carrots)

1/4 cup low-sodium chicken broth, 1 tablespoon olive oil, 1 teaspoon minced garlic,

1/2 teaspoon dried thyme, Salt and pepper to taste.

Instructions:

Preheat the oven to 375°F (190°C).

Season the chicken breast with salt, pepper, and dried thyme.

In a baking dish, arrange the seasoned chicken breast and mixed vegetables.

In a small bowl, whisk together chicken broth, olive oil, and minced garlic.

Pour the mixture over the chicken and vegetables in the baking dish.

Cover the baking dish with foil and bake in the preheated oven for 25-30 minutes, or until the chicken is cooked through and vegetables are tender.

Serve hot as a comforting and nutritious dinner option.

Nutritional Facts (per serving):

Protein: 25g

Fiber: 3g

Sodium: 200mg

Tips:

Use boneless, skinless chicken thighs as an alternative to chicken breast.

Recipe 6: Quinoa Stuffed Bell Peppers

Prep Time: 15 minutes

Cook Time: 30 minutes

Serving Size: 1 stuffed pepper

Ingredients:

2 large bell peppers, halved and seeds removed, 1 cup cooked quinoa

1/2 cup black beans, drained and rinsed, 1/2 cup diced tomatoes

1/4 cup diced red onion, 1/4 cup shredded low-fat cheese

1 teaspoon olive oil, 1 teaspoon minced garlic, 1 teaspoon chili powder, Salt and pepper to taste

Instructions:

Preheat the oven to 375°F (190°C).

In a skillet, heat olive oil over medium heat. Add minced garlic and sauté until fragrant.

Add diced red onion and cook until softened, about 2-3 minutes.

Stir in cooked quinoa, black beans, diced tomatoes, chili powder, salt, and pepper. Cook for an additional 2-3 minutes.

Spoon the quinoa mixture into halved bell peppers.

Place stuffed peppers in a baking dish, cover with foil, and bake for 25-30 minutes.

Remove foil, sprinkle shredded cheese over the stuffed peppers, and bake for an additional 5 minutes, or until cheese is melted and bubbly.

Nutritional Facts (per serving):

Protein: 8g

Fat: 5g

Sodium: 200mg

Tips:

Customize with your favorite vegetables or protein sources.

Recipe 7: Turkey Meatball and Vegetable Soup

Prep Time: 15 minutes

Cook Time: 25 minutes

Serving Size: 1 cup

Ingredients:

4 ounces lean ground turkey, 4 cups low-sodium chicken broth, 1 carrot, diced

1 celery stalk, diced, 1/2 onion, diced, 1 teaspoon minced garlic

1 teaspoon dried Italian herbs, Salt and pepper to taste

Instructions:

In a mixing bowl, combine lean ground turkey with dried Italian herbs, salt, and pepper. Roll into small meatballs.

In a large pot, heat olive oil over medium heat. Add minced garlic and cook until fragrant.

Add diced carrot, celery, and onion to the pot and cook until softened, about 5 minutes.

Pour in low-sodium chicken broth and bring to a simmer.

Gently drop meatballs into the simmering broth and cook for 10-15 minutes until cooked through.

Nutritional Facts (per serving):

Protein: 15g

Fat: 6g

Sodium: 200mg

Tips:

Garnish with chopped fresh parsley or grated Parmesan cheese before serving.

Recipe 8: Baked Lemon Herb Chicken

Prep Time: 10 minutes

Cook Time: 25 minutes

Serving Size: 1 chicken breast

Ingredients:

1 boneless, skinless chicken breast, 1 tablespoon olive oil, 1 tablespoon lemon juice

1 teaspoon dried herbs (such as thyme or rosemary), Salt and pepper to taste

Instructions:

Preheat the oven to 375°F (190°C).

In a small bowl, whisk together olive oil, lemon juice, dried herbs, salt, and pepper.

Place the chicken breast in a baking dish and brush with the lemon herb mixture.

Bake in the preheated oven for 20-25 minutes, or until chicken is cooked through and juices run clear.

Nutritional Facts (per serving):

Protein: 25g

Fat: 8g

Sodium: 70mg

Tips:

Garnish with lemon slices or fresh herbs before serving.

Recipe 9: Vegetable and Tofu Stir-Fry

Prep Time: 15 minutes

Cook Time: 10 minutes

Serving Size: 1 cup

Ingredients:

4 ounces firm tofu, cubed, 1 cup mixed vegetables (such as bell peppers, snap peas, and broccoli)

2 tablespoons low-sodium soy sauce, 1 tablespoon olive oil

1 teaspoon minced garlic, 1 teaspoon minced ginger

Instructions:

Heat olive oil in a large skillet or wok over medium-high heat.

Add minced garlic and ginger, and sauté for 1 minute until fragrant.

Add cubed tofu to the skillet and cook until lightly browned on all sides.

Add mixed vegetables to the skillet and stir-fry for 3-4 minutes until tender-crisp.

Drizzle low-sodium soy sauce over the tofu and vegetables, and toss to combine.

Cook for another minute until heated through.

Nutritional Facts (per serving):

Protein: 10g

Fat: 8g

Sodium: 300mg

Tips:

Add a splash of rice vinegar or lime juice for extra flavor.

Recipe 10: Spaghetti Squash with Marinara Sauce

Prep Time: 10 minutes

Cook Time: 40 minutes

Serving Size: 1 cup

Ingredients:

1 medium spaghetti squash, 1 cup low-sodium marinara sauce

1 tablespoon olive oil, 1 teaspoon minced garlic, Salt and pepper to taste

Instructions:

Preheat the oven to 375°F (190°C).

Cut the spaghetti squash in half lengthwise and remove the seeds.

Drizzle olive oil over the cut sides of the squash and season with minced garlic, salt, and pepper.

Place the squash halves cut side down on a baking sheet lined with parchment paper.

Bake in the preheated oven for 30-40 minutes, or until the squash is tender and easily pierced with a fork.

Use a fork to scrape the flesh of the squash into spaghetti-like strands.

Nutritional Facts (per serving):

Protein: 2g

Fiber: 5g

Sodium: 150mg

Tips:

Add cooked lean ground turkey or tofu for extra protein.

Chapter 6: Snack and Appetizers Recipes

Recipe 1: Cucumber and Cottage Cheese Bites

Prep Time: 10 minutes

Serving Size: 2 cucumber slices with cottage cheese

Ingredients:

1 cucumber, sliced

1/4 cup low-fat cottage cheese, Fresh dill or parsley for garnish (optional).

Instructions:

Place cucumber slices on a serving platter.

Top each cucumber slice with a small spoonful of cottage cheese.

Garnish with fresh dill or parsley if desired.

Serve immediately as a refreshing and protein-rich snack.

Nutritional Facts (per serving):

Protein: 3g

Fiber: 1g

Sodium: 80mg

Tips:

Add a sprinkle of black pepper or paprika for extra flavor.

Recipe 2: Hummus and Veggie Platter

Prep Time: 10 minutes

Serving Size: 2 tablespoons hummus with veggie sticks

Ingredients:

1/2 cup hummus (store-bought or homemade)

Assorted vegetable sticks (carrots, cucumber, bell peppers, celery)

Instructions:

Arrange hummus in a small bowl in the center of a serving platter.

Surround the hummus with assorted vegetable sticks.

Serve immediately as a nutritious and fiber-rich snack.

Nutritional Facts (per serving):

Protein: 3g

Fiber: 3g

Sodium: 150mg

Tips:

Opt for low-sodium hummus if available.

Recipe 3: Greek Yogurt Parfait

Prep Time: 5 minutes

Serving Size: 1 parfait

Ingredients:

1/2 cup plain Greek yogurt

1/4 cup fresh berries (such as strawberries, blueberries, raspberries)

1 tablespoon chopped nuts (such as almonds or walnuts)

Instructions:

In a glass or serving bowl, layer Greek yogurt, fresh berries, and chopped nuts.

Drizzle with honey if desired.

Serve immediately as a protein-packed and antioxidant-rich snack.

Nutritional Facts (per serving):

Protein: 15g

Fiber: 3g

Sodium: 50mg

Tips:

Use unsweetened Greek yogurt to reduce added sugars.

Recipe 4: Rice Cake with Almond Butter and Banana Slices

Prep Time: 5 minutes

Serving Size: 1 rice cake with almond butter and banana slices

Ingredients:

1 rice cake

1 tablespoon almond butter (or any nut butter)

1/2 small banana, sliced

Instructions:

Spread almond butter evenly on top of the rice cake.

Arrange banana slices on top of the almond butter.

Serve immediately as a quick and satisfying snack.

Nutritional Facts (per serving):

Protein: 3g

Fiber: 2g

Sodium: 50mg

Tips:

Choose unsalted rice cakes to reduce sodium intake.

Recipe 5: Caprese Skewers

Prep Time: 10 minutes

Serving Size: 2 skewers

Ingredients:

Cherry tomatoes

Fresh mozzarella balls

Fresh basil leaves

Instructions:

Thread cherry tomatoes, fresh mozzarella balls, and basil leaves onto small skewers.

Arrange the skewers on a serving platter.

Drizzle with balsamic glaze if desired.

Serve immediately as a flavorful and low-calorie snack.

Nutritional Facts (per serving):

Protein: 5g

Fiber: 1g

Sodium: 100mg

Tips:

Sprinkle with a pinch of sea salt before serving for added flavor.

Recipe 6: Egg Salad Lettuce Wraps

Prep Time: 15 minutes

Serving Size: 2 lettuce wraps

Ingredients:

2 hard-boiled eggs, chopped, 2 tablespoons plain Greek yogurt

1 teaspoon Dijon mustard, 1 teaspoon chopped fresh dill

Salt and pepper to taste, 4 large lettuce leaves (such as romaine or butter lettuce).

Instructions:

In a mixing bowl, combine chopped hard-boiled eggs, Greek yogurt, Dijon mustard, chopped dill, salt, and pepper.

Mix until well combined.

Spoon the egg salad mixture onto lettuce leaves.

Roll up the lettuce leaves to form wraps.

Serve immediately as a protein-rich and low-carb snack.

Nutritional Facts (per serving):

Protein: 10g

Fiber: 1g

Sodium: 150mg

Tips:

Sprinkle with paprika or black pepper before serving.

Recipe 7: Edamame Hummus

Prep Time: 10 minutes

Serving Size: 2 tablespoons

Ingredients:

1 cup shelled edamame (thawed if using frozen)

2 tablespoons tahini, 1 tablespoon olive oil

1 tablespoon lemon juice, 1 clove garlic, minced, Salt and pepper to taste.

Instructions:

In a food processor, combine shelled edamame, tahini, olive oil, lemon juice, minced garlic, salt, and pepper.

Blend until smooth and creamy, scraping down the sides as needed.

If the hummus is too thick, add a tablespoon of water at a time until desired consistency is reached.

Serve with vegetable sticks or whole grain crackers as a nutritious and protein-packed snack.

Nutritional Facts (per serving):

Protein: 4g

Fiber: 2g

Sodium: 70mg

Tips:

Add a pinch of cumin or smoked paprika for extra flavor.

Recipe 8: Zucchini Fritters

Prep Time: 15 minutes

Cook Time: 15 minutes

Serving Size: 2 fritters

Ingredients:

1 medium zucchini, grated, 1/4 cup grated Parmesan cheese

2 tablespoons whole wheat flour, 1 egg, beaten

1 clove garlic, minced, Salt and pepper to taste, Olive oil for frying.

Instructions:

Place grated zucchini in a clean kitchen towel and squeeze out excess moisture.

In a mixing bowl, combine grated zucchini, Parmesan cheese, whole wheat flour, beaten egg, minced garlic, salt, and pepper.

Heat olive oil in a skillet over medium heat.

Drop spoonfuls of the zucchini mixture into the skillet and flatten with the back of a spoon to form fritters.

Cook for 3-4 minutes on each side until golden brown and cooked through.

Serve hot as a flavorful and vegetable-packed appetizer.

Nutritional Facts (per serving):

Protein: 5g

Fiber: 1g

Sodium: 120mg

Tips:

Serve with a dollop of Greek yogurt or tzatziki sauce for dipping.

Recipe 9: Stuffed Mini Bell Peppers

Prep Time: 15 minutes

Cook Time: 15 minutes

Serving Size: 2 stuffed peppers

Ingredients:

6 mini bell peppers, halved and seeds removed

1/2 cup low-fat cream cheese, 1/4 cup chopped fresh herbs (such as parsley or chives)

1 tablespoon lemon juice, Salt and pepper to taste.

Instructions:

Preheat the oven to 375°F (190°C).

In a mixing bowl, combine low-fat cream cheese, chopped fresh herbs, lemon juice, salt, and pepper.

Spoon the cream cheese mixture into halved mini bell peppers.

Place stuffed peppers on a baking sheet lined with parchment paper.

Bake in the preheated oven for 12-15 minutes, or until peppers are tender and cheese is melted.

Nutritional Facts (per serving):

Protein: 3g

Fiber: 1g

Sodium: 80mg

Tips:

Garnish with additional chopped herbs before serving.

Recipe 10: Baked Eggplant Chips

Prep Time: 10 minutes

Cook Time: 20 minutes

Serving Size: 1/2 cup

Ingredients:

1 medium eggplant, thinly sliced into rounds

2 tablespoons olive oil, 1 teaspoon Italian seasoning, Salt and pepper to taste

Instructions:

Preheat the oven to 400°F (200°C).

Place eggplant slices in a single layer on a baking sheet lined with parchment paper.

Drizzle olive oil over the eggplant slices and sprinkle with Italian seasoning, salt, and pepper.

Bake in the preheated oven for 15-20 minutes, or until eggplant slices are golden brown and crispy.

Nutritional Facts (per serving):

Protein: 1g

Fat: 7g

Sodium: 150mg

Tips:

Sprinkle with grated Parmesan cheese before baking for extra flavor.

Chapter 7: Soups and Salads

Recipe 1: Minestrone Soup

Prep Time: 15 minutes

Cook Time: 30 minutes

Serving Size: 1 cup

Ingredients:

4 cups low-sodium vegetable broth

1 can (14 oz) low-sodium diced tomatoes, 1/2 cup diced carrots, 1/2 cup diced celery

1/2 cup diced zucchini, 1/2 cup cooked kidney beans

1/2 cup cooked whole grain pasta (such as penne or fusilli), 1 teaspoon dried Italian herbs, Salt and pepper to taste.

Instructions:

In a large pot, bring vegetable broth to a simmer over medium heat.

Add diced tomatoes, carrots, celery, zucchini, and dried Italian herbs to the pot.

Simmer for 20-25 minutes, or until vegetables are tender.

Stir in cooked kidney beans and pasta.

Season with salt and pepper to taste.

Serve hot as a hearty and nutritious soup option.

Nutritional Facts (per serving):

Protein: 5g

Fat: 1g

Sodium: 200mg

Tips:

Garnish with chopped fresh parsley or grated Parmesan cheese before serving.

Recipe 2: Chicken and Vegetable Soup

Prep Time: 15 minutes

Cook Time: 30 minutes

Serving Size: 1 cup

Ingredients:

4 cups low-sodium chicken broth, 1 boneless, skinless chicken breast

1 carrot, diced, 1 celery stalk, diced, 1/2 onion, diced

1 teaspoon minced garlic, 1 teaspoon dried thyme, Salt and pepper to taste

Instructions:

In a large pot, bring chicken broth to a simmer over medium heat.

Add chicken breast, diced carrot, celery, onion, minced garlic, and dried thyme to the pot.

Simmer for 20-25 minutes, or until chicken is cooked through and vegetables are tender.

Remove chicken breast from the pot and shred with two forks.

Return shredded chicken to the pot and season with salt and pepper to taste.

Serve hot as a comforting and protein-rich soup option.

Nutritional Facts (per serving):

Protein: 15g

Fat: 3g

Sodium: 150mg

Tips:

Add cooked brown rice or quinoa for extra texture and fiber.

Recipe 3: Mixed Greens Salad with Lemon Vinaigrette

Prep Time: 10 minutes

Serving Size: 1 cup

Ingredients:

2 cups mixed salad greens (such as spinach, arugula, and romaine)

1/4 cup cherry tomatoes, halved, 1/4 cup cucumber, sliced

1/4 cup shredded carrots, 1 tablespoon lemon juice

1 tablespoon olive oil, 1 teaspoon Dijon mustard, Salt and pepper to taste

Instructions:

In a large salad bowl, combine mixed greens, cherry tomatoes, cucumber, and shredded carrots.

In a small bowl, whisk together lemon juice, olive oil, Dijon mustard, salt, and pepper to make the vinaigrette.

Drizzle the vinaigrette over the salad and toss to coat evenly.

Serve immediately as a refreshing and nutrient-rich salad option.

Nutritional Facts (per serving):

Protein: 1g

Fat: 4g

Sodium: 50mg

Tips:

Add sliced avocado or toasted nuts for extra flavor and healthy fats.

Recipe 4: Tomato Basil Soup

Prep Time: 10 minutes

Cook Time: 25 minutes

Serving Size: 1 cup

Ingredients:

4 cups low-sodium vegetable broth, 1 can (14 oz) low-sodium diced tomatoes

1/2 onion, diced, 2 cloves garlic, minced, 1/4 cup chopped fresh basil

1 tablespoon olive oil, Salt and pepper to taste

Instructions:

In a large pot, heat olive oil over medium heat.

Add diced onion and minced garlic to the pot and sauté until softened.

Stir in diced tomatoes (with juices) and chopped fresh basil.

Add vegetable broth to the pot and bring to a simmer.

Simmer for 15-20 minutes, allowing flavors to meld together.

Use an immersion blender to blend the soup until smooth (or transfer to a blender and blend in batches).

Nutritional Facts (per serving):

Protein: 2g

Fat: 3g

Sodium: 200mg

Tips:

Garnish with a drizzle of olive oil and a sprinkle of chopped fresh basil before serving.

Recipe 5: Spinach and Strawberry Salad

Prep Time: 10 minutes

Serving Size: 1 cup

Ingredients:

2 cups baby spinach leaves, 1/2 cup sliced strawberries

1/4 cup crumbled feta cheese, 2 tablespoons chopped walnuts

1 tablespoon balsamic vinegar, 1 teaspoon olive oil, 1 teaspoon honey

Instructions:

In a large salad bowl, combine baby spinach leaves, sliced strawberries, crumbled feta cheese, and chopped walnuts.

In a small bowl, whisk together balsamic vinegar, olive oil, and honey to make the dressing.

Drizzle the dressing over the salad and toss to coat evenly.

Serve immediately as a vibrant and antioxidant-rich salad option.

Nutritional Facts (per serving):

Protein: 3g

Fat: 6g

Sodium: 120mg

Tips:

Substitute goat cheese or blue cheese for feta cheese if desired.

Recipe 6: Lentil and Vegetable Soup

Prep Time: 15 minutes

Cook Time: 40 minutes

Serving Size: 1 cup

Ingredients:

1 cup dried green lentils, rinsed and drained, 4 cups low-sodium vegetable broth

1 carrot, diced, 1 celery stalk, diced, 1/2 onion, diced

1 teaspoon minced garlic, 1 teaspoon ground cumin, 1/2 teaspoon smoked paprika

Instructions:

In a large pot, combine dried lentils and vegetable broth.

Bring to a boil over medium-high heat, then reduce heat to low and simmer for 20 minutes.

Add diced carrot, celery, onion, minced garlic, ground cumin, smoked paprika, salt, and pepper to the pot.

Continue to simmer for an additional 15-20 minutes, or until lentils and vegetables are tender.

Serve hot as a protein-packed and fiber-rich soup option.

Nutritional Facts (per serving):

Protein: 10g

Fat: 1g

Sodium: 200mg

Tips:

Add a squeeze of lemon juice before serving for a burst of freshness.

Recipe 7: Quinoa and Black Bean Salad

Prep Time: 15 minutes

Cook Time: 15 minutes

Serving Size: 1 cup

Ingredients:

1/2 cup quinoa, rinsed and drained, 1 cup water

1 can (15 oz) low-sodium black beans, rinsed and drained, 1/2 cup diced bell pepper (any color)

1/4 cup chopped fresh cilantro, 2 tablespoons lime juice

1 tablespoon olive oil, 1 teaspoon ground cumin, Salt and pepper to taste

Instructions:

In a small saucepan, combine quinoa and water.

Bring to a boil, then reduce heat to low and simmer for 15 minutes, or until quinoa is tender and water is absorbed.

In a large bowl, combine cooked quinoa, black beans, diced bell pepper, chopped cilantro, lime juice, olive oil, ground cumin, salt, and pepper.

Toss to combine all ingredients evenly.

Serve chilled or at room temperature as a protein-rich and nutrient-dense salad option.

Nutritional Facts (per serving):

Calories: 180

Protein: 8g

Carbohydrates: 28g

Fat: 4g

Fiber: 7g

Sodium: 200mg

Tips:

Drizzle with a balsamic vinaigrette for additional tanginess.

Recipe 8: Butternut Squash Soup

Prep Time: 15 minutes

Cook Time: 30 minutes

Serving Size: 1 cup

Ingredients:

1 small butternut squash, peeled, seeded, and diced

1 carrot, diced, 1 celery stalk, diced, 1/2 onion, diced

2 cups low-sodium vegetable broth, 1/2 teaspoon ground cinnamon, 1/4 teaspoon ground nutmeg

Instructions:

In a large pot, combine diced butternut squash, carrot, celery, onion, and vegetable broth.

Bring to a boil, then reduce heat to low and simmer for 20-25 minutes, or until vegetables are tender.

Use an immersion blender to blend the soup until smooth (or transfer to a blender and blend in batches).

Stir in ground cinnamon and ground nutmeg.

Season with salt and pepper to taste.

Serve hot as a creamy and comforting soup option.

Nutritional Facts (per serving):

Protein: 2g

Fat: 1g

Sodium: 200mg

Tips:

Substitute sweet potatoes for butternut squash for a similar flavor profile.

Recipe 9: Chickpea and Avocado Salad

Prep Time: 15 minutes

Serving Size: 1 cup

Ingredients:

1 can (15 oz) low-sodium chickpeas, rinsed and drained

1 avocado, diced, 1/4 cup diced red onion, 1/4 cup chopped fresh cilantro

2 tablespoons lime juice, 1 tablespoon olive oil, 1/2 teaspoon ground cumin

Instructions:

In a large bowl, combine chickpeas, diced avocado, diced red onion, chopped cilantro, lime juice, olive oil, ground cumin, salt, and pepper.

Gently toss to combine all ingredients evenly.

Serve chilled or at room temperature as a protein-rich and creamy salad option.

Nutritional Facts (per serving):

Protein: 6g

Fiber: 8g

Sodium: 150mg

Tips:

Add diced cherry tomatoes or bell peppers for extra color and flavor.

Recipe 10: Cucumber and Tomato Salad

Prep Time: 10 minutes

Serving Size: 1 cup

Ingredients:

1 cucumber, diced

1 cup cherry tomatoes, halved, 1/4 cup diced red onion

2 tablespoons chopped fresh parsley, 1 tablespoon apple cider vinegar

1 tablespoon olive oil, 1 teaspoon honey

Instructions:

In a large bowl, combine diced cucumber, halved cherry tomatoes, diced red onion, and chopped parsley.

In a small bowl, whisk together apple cider vinegar, olive oil, and honey to make the dressing.

Drizzle the dressing over the salad and toss to coat evenly.

Serve immediately as a refreshing and hydrating salad option.

Nutritional Facts (per serving):

Protein: 1g

Fat: 3g

Sodium: 20mg

Tips:

Serve with a sprinkle of black pepper or a pinch of red pepper flakes for added heat.

Chapter 8: Desserts and Treats

Recipe 1: Baked Apples with Cinnamon

Prep Time: 10 minutes

Cook Time: 30 minutes

Serving Size: 1 apple

Ingredients:

2 apples, cored, 1 tablespoon lemon juice

1 teaspoon ground cinnamon, 1 tablespoon honey (optional)

Instructions:

Preheat the oven to 375°F (190°C).

Core the apples and place them in a baking dish.

Drizzle lemon juice over the apples and sprinkle with ground cinnamon.

Bake in the preheated oven for 25-30 minutes, or until apples are tender.

Serve warm as a comforting and naturally sweet dessert option.

Nutritional Facts (per serving):

Protein: 0g

Fiber: 4g

Sodium: 0mg

Tips:

Experiment with different apple varieties such as Granny Smith or Fuji.

Recipe 2: Berry Parfait

Prep Time: 10 minutes

Serving Size: 1 parfait

Ingredients:

1/2 cup low-fat Greek yogurt

1/4 cup mixed berries (such as strawberries, blueberries, and raspberries)

2 tablespoons granola, 1 teaspoon honey (optional)

Instructions:

In a glass or serving dish, layer low-fat Greek yogurt, mixed berries, and granola.

Optionally, drizzle honey over the parfait for added sweetness.

Repeat the layers until all ingredients are used, ending with a layer of granola on top.

Serve immediately as a light and protein-rich dessert or snack option.

Nutritional Facts (per serving):

Protein: 8g

Fat: 2g

Sodium: 60mg

Tips:

Use unsweetened granola to reduce added sugars.

Recipe 3: Chia Seed Pudding

Prep Time: 5 minutes (+ chilling time)

Serving Size: 1/2 cup

Ingredients:

2 tablespoons chia seeds, 1/2 cup unsweetened almond milk (or any milk of choice)

1/4 teaspoon vanilla extract, 1 teaspoon honey (optional)

Instructions:

In a small bowl or jar, combine chia seeds, unsweetened almond milk, vanilla extract, and honey (if using).

Stir well to combine all ingredients.

Cover and refrigerate for at least 2 hours or overnight, until the mixture thickens into a pudding-like consistency.

Serve chilled as a nutritious and omega-3-rich dessert option.

Nutritional Facts (per serving):

Protein: 3g

Fat: 4g

Sodium: 60mg

Tips:

Top with fresh fruit, chopped nuts, or a sprinkle of cinnamon before serving.

Recipe 4: Frozen Banana Bites

Prep Time: 10 minutes (+ freezing time)

Serving Size: 2 banana bites

Ingredients:

1 ripe banana, peeled and sliced, 2 tablespoons unsweetened peanut butter (or any nut or seed butter)

1/4 cup dark chocolate chips, 1 teaspoon coconut oil

Instructions:

Spread peanut butter onto half of the banana slices and top with the remaining slices to make sandwiches.

Place banana sandwiches on a baking sheet lined with parchment paper.

In a microwave-safe bowl, combine dark chocolate chips and coconut oil. Microwave in 30-second intervals, stirring in between, until chocolate is melted and smooth.

Dip each banana sandwich into the melted chocolate, coating evenly.

Return chocolate-covered banana sandwiches to the baking sheet and freeze for at least 1 hour, or until chocolate is set.

Serve frozen as a creamy and indulgent dessert option.

Nutritional Facts (per serving):

Protein: 2g

Fat: 7g

Fiber: 2g

Tips:

Sprinkle chopped nuts or shredded coconut over the chocolate coating before freezing.

Recipe 5: Vanilla Rice Pudding

Prep Time: 5 minutes

Cook Time: 25 minutes

Serving Size: 1/2 cup

Ingredients:

1/4 cup Arborio rice, 2 cups unsweetened almond milk (or any milk of choice)

2 tablespoons honey (or sweetener of choice), 1 teaspoon vanilla extract

Instructions:

In a medium saucepan, combine Arborio rice and unsweetened almond milk.

Bring to a boil over medium-high heat, then reduce heat to low and simmer for 20-25 minutes, stirring occasionally, until rice is tender and mixture is creamy.

Stir in honey and vanilla extract.

Continue to cook for an additional 2-3 minutes, until pudding thickens slightly.

Remove from heat and let cool slightly before serving.

Serve warm or chilled as a comforting and classic dessert option.

Nutritional Facts (per serving):

Protein: 2g

Fiber: 1g

Sodium: 80mg

Tips:

Add a sprinkle of ground cinnamon or nutmeg for extra flavor.

Recipe 6: Coconut Yogurt Parfait

Prep Time: 10 minutes

Serving Size: 1 parfait

Ingredients:

1/2 cup unsweetened coconut yogurt, 1/4 cup diced pineapple

1 tablespoon shredded coconut, 1 tablespoon chopped almonds

Instructions:

In a glass or serving dish, layer unsweetened coconut yogurt, diced pineapple, shredded coconut, and chopped almonds.

Repeat the layers until all ingredients are used.

Serve immediately as a tropical and dairy-free dessert option.

Nutritional Facts (per serving):

Protein: 3g

Fat: 11g

Sodium: 15mg

Tips:

Use fresh or frozen fruit of your choice for variation.

Recipe 7: No-Bake Energy Bites

Prep Time: 10 minutes (+ chilling time)

Serving Size: 2 bites

Ingredients:

1/2 cup rolled oats, 1/4 cup natural peanut butter

2 tablespoons honey, 2 tablespoons ground flaxseed, 1/4 cup mini chocolate chips

Instructions:

In a mixing bowl, combine rolled oats, natural peanut butter, honey, ground flaxseed, and mini chocolate chips.

Stir until all ingredients are evenly incorporated.

Roll the mixture into small bite-sized balls and place them on a baking sheet lined with parchment paper.

Chill in the refrigerator for at least 30 minutes, or until firm.

Serve chilled as a protein-packed and energy-boosting snack or dessert option.

Nutritional Facts (per serving):

Protein: 4g

Fat: 6g

Fiber: 2g

Sodium: 20mg

Tips:

Add chopped nuts or dried fruit for extra texture and flavor.

Recipe 8: Peach Frozen Yogurt

Prep Time: 5 minutes (+ freezing time)

Serving Size: 1/2 cup

Ingredients:

1 cup frozen peach slices

1/2 cup unsweetened Greek yogurt

1 tablespoon honey (optional)

Instructions:

In a blender or food processor, combine frozen peach slices, unsweetened Greek yogurt, and honey (if using).

Blend until smooth and creamy.

Transfer the mixture to a freezer-safe container and freeze for 2-3 hours, or until firm.

Serve frozen as a refreshing and calcium-rich dessert option.

Nutritional Facts (per serving):

Protein: 4g

Fiber: 2g

Sodium: 20mg

Tips:

Substitute other frozen fruits such as berries or mango for variation.

Recipe 9: Chocolate Avocado Mousse

Prep Time: 10 minutes

Serving Size: 1/4 cup

Ingredients:

1 ripe avocado, peeled and pitted, 2 tablespoons cocoa powder

2 tablespoons honey, 1/2 teaspoon vanilla extract

Instructions:

In a blender or food processor, combine ripe avocado, cocoa powder, honey, and vanilla extract.

Blend until smooth and creamy.

Transfer the mixture to serving dishes and refrigerate for at least 30 minutes before serving.

Serve chilled as a rich and indulgent dessert option.

Nutritional Facts (per serving):

Protein: 2g

Fiber: 5g

Sodium: 0mg

Tips:

Top with fresh berries or a dollop of whipped cream if desired.

Recipe 10: Frozen Grape Skewers

Prep Time: 10 minutes (+ freezing time)

Serving Size: 1 skewer

Ingredients:

Seedless grapes (any variety)

Instructions:

Thread seedless grapes onto wooden skewers, leaving space between each grape.

Place the grape skewers on a baking sheet lined with parchment paper.

Freeze for at least 2 hours, or until grapes are firm.

Serve frozen as a simple and refreshing dessert or snack option.

Nutritional Facts (per serving):

Carbohydrates: 8g

Fiber: 1g

Sodium: 0mg

Tips:

Use a variety of grape colors for a colorful presentation.

Chapter 9: Herbal Tea Recipes for kidney support

Recipe 1: Dandelion Root Tea

Prep Time: 5 minutes

Serving Size: 1 cup

Ingredients:

1 teaspoon dried dandelion root

1 cup water

Instructions:

Boil water in a small saucepan.

Add dried dandelion root to the boiling water.

Reduce heat to low and let simmer for 5 minutes.

Strain the tea into a cup and discard the dandelion root.

Serve hot and enjoy the kidney-supporting benefits of dandelion root tea.

Tips:

Add a slice of lemon or a dash of honey for extra flavor if desired.

Recipe 2: Nettle Leaf Tea

Prep Time: 5 minutes

Serving Size: 1 cup

Ingredients:

1 teaspoon dried nettle leaves

1 cup water

Instructions:

Bring water to a boil in a small saucepan.

Add dried nettle leaves to the boiling water.

Reduce heat to low and let simmer for 5 minutes.

Strain the tea into a cup and discard the nettle leaves.

Serve hot and enjoy the kidney-supporting benefits of nettle leaf tea.

Tips:

Nettle leaf tea can have a mild, earthy flavor. Add a slice of lemon or a teaspoon of honey to enhance the taste.

Recipe 3: Marshmallow Root Tea

Prep Time: 5 minutes

Serving Size: 1 cup

Ingredients:

1 teaspoon dried marshmallow root

1 cup water

Instructions:

Bring water to a boil in a small saucepan.

Add dried marshmallow root to the boiling water.

Reduce heat to low and let simmer for 5 minutes.

Strain the tea into a cup and discard the marshmallow root.

Serve hot and enjoy the kidney-supporting benefits of marshmallow root tea.

Tips:

Marshmallow root tea has a mild, slightly sweet flavor. Enjoy it as is or add a touch of honey for extra sweetness.

Recipe 4: Corn Silk Tea

Prep Time: 5 minutes

Serving Size: 1 cup

Ingredients:

1 teaspoon dried corn silk

1 cup water

Instructions:

Bring water to a boil in a small saucepan.

Add dried corn silk to the boiling water.

Reduce heat to low and let simmer for 5 minutes.

Strain the tea into a cup and discard the corn silk.

Serve hot and enjoy the kidney-supporting benefits of corn silk tea.

Tips:

Corn silk tea has a mild, slightly sweet flavor. Add a splash of lemon juice or a sprinkle of cinnamon for extra flavor.

Drink 1-2 cups daily for kidney support.

Recipe 5: Ginger Turmeric Tea

Prep Time: 5 minutes

Serving Size: 1 cup

Ingredients:

1 teaspoon grated fresh ginger

1/2 teaspoon ground turmeric

1 cup water

Instructions:

In a small saucepan, bring water to a boil.

Add grated ginger and ground turmeric to the boiling water.

Reduce heat to low and let simmer for 5 minutes.

Strain the tea into a cup.

Serve hot and enjoy the kidney-supporting benefits of ginger turmeric tea.

Tips:

Ginger turmeric tea has a warm and spicy flavor. Add a touch of honey or a slice of lemon for sweetness and extra flavor.

Drink 1-2 cups daily for kidney support.

Chapter 10: Low-Sodium Infused water Recipes

Recipe 1: Cucumber Mint Infused Water

Prep Time: 5 minutes

Serving Size: 1 glass

Ingredients:

1/2 cucumber, sliced

4-5 fresh mint leaves

1 cup water

Instructions:

Place cucumber slices and mint leaves in a glass or pitcher.

Fill the container with water.

Let it sit in the refrigerator for at least 1 hour to allow the flavors to infuse.

Serve chilled over ice and enjoy!

Tips:

For a stronger flavor, muddle the mint leaves slightly before adding water.

You can refill the container with water a couple of times before replacing the cucumber and mint.

Recipe 2: Citrus Basil Infused Water

Prep Time: 5 minutes

Serving Size: 1 glass

Ingredients:

1/2 orange, sliced, 1/2 lemon, sliced

2-3 fresh basil leaves, 1 cup water

Instructions:

Place orange slices, lemon slices, and basil leaves in a glass or pitcher.

Fill the container with water.

Allow it to sit in the refrigerator for at least 1 hour to infuse the flavors.

Serve chilled over ice and enjoy the refreshing taste!

Tips:

Experiment with different citrus fruits like lime or grapefruit for variation.

Garnish with a sprig of basil before serving for an elegant touch.

Recipe 3: Berry Rosemary Infused Water

Prep Time: 5 minutes

Serving Size: 1 glass

Ingredients:

1/4 cup mixed berries (such as strawberries, blueberries, raspberries)

1 small sprig of fresh rosemary

1 cup water

Instructions:

Place mixed berries and rosemary sprig in a glass or pitcher.

Fill the container with water.

Let it infuse in the refrigerator for at least 1 hour.

Serve chilled and enjoy the delightful combination of flavors!

Tips:

Gently crush the berries with a spoon before adding water to release their juices.

Use frozen berries if fresh ones are not available for a similar flavor.

Recipe 4: Pineapple Ginger Infused Water

Prep Time: 5 minutes

Serving Size: 1 glass

Ingredients:

1/2 cup pineapple chunks

2-3 slices of fresh ginger, 1 cup water

Instructions:

Place pineapple chunks and ginger slices in a glass or pitcher.

Fill the container with water.

Allow it to infuse in the refrigerator for at least 1 hour.

Serve chilled over ice for a refreshing tropical flavor!

Tips:

Add a squeeze of lime juice for an extra burst of citrus flavor.

Use a muddler to lightly crush the ginger slices before adding water for a stronger taste.

Recipe 5: Watermelon Basil Infused Water

Prep Time: 5 minutes

Serving Size: 1 glass

Ingredients:

1/2 cup watermelon cubes

2-3 fresh basil leaves, 1 cup water

Instructions:

Place watermelon cubes and basil leaves in a glass or pitcher.

Fill the container with water.

Let it infuse in the refrigerator for at least 1 hour.

Serve chilled over ice and enjoy the refreshing and hydrating beverage!

Tips:

For a twist, add a splash of lime juice or a few cucumber slices to enhance the flavor.

Use seedless watermelon for easier preparation and serving.

Chapter 11: 28-Day Meal plan

Day 1:

Breakfast: Oatmeal with Berries

Prep Time: 5 minutes

Ingredients:

1/2 cup rolled oats, 1 cup water

1/4 cup mixed berries, 1 tablespoon chopped almonds

Instructions:

In a saucepan, bring water to a boil.

Add rolled oats and cook until thickened, stirring occasionally.

Serve topped with mixed berries and chopped almonds.

Calories: 250

Lunch: Grilled Chicken Salad

Prep Time: 15 minutes

Ingredients:

3 oz grilled chicken breast, Mixed salad greens

1/4 cup cherry tomatoes, halved, 1/4 cucumber, sliced, 1 tablespoon balsamic vinaigrette

Instructions:

Arrange salad greens on a plate.

Top with grilled chicken, cherry tomatoes, and cucumber slices.

Drizzle with balsamic vinaigrette.

Calories: 300

Dinner: Baked Salmon with Steamed Vegetables

Prep Time: 20 minutes

Ingredients:

4 oz salmon fillet, 1/2 cup broccoli florets

1/2 cup carrots, sliced, 1 teaspoon olive oil, Lemon slices

Instructions:

Preheat oven to 375°F (190°C).

Place salmon on a baking sheet lined with parchment paper. Top with lemon slices.

Arrange broccoli and carrots around the salmon. Drizzle with olive oil.

Bake for 15-20 minutes or until salmon is cooked through and vegetables are tender.

Calories: 350

Snack: Greek Yogurt with Honey

Prep Time: 5 minutes

Ingredients:

1/2 cup plain Greek yogurt

1 teaspoon honey

Instructions:

Place Greek yogurt in a bowl.

Drizzle with honey.

Calories: 120

Day 2:

Breakfast: Spinach and Mushroom Omelette

Prep Time: 10 minutes

Ingredients:

2 eggs, 1/4 cup spinach, chopped

1/4 cup mushrooms, sliced, 1 tablespoon shredded mozzarella cheese, Salt and pepper to taste

Instructions:

In a bowl, beat eggs until frothy. Season with salt and pepper.

Heat a non-stick skillet over medium heat. Add spinach and mushrooms, cook until softened.

Pour beaten eggs over the vegetables. Cook until the edges are set, then sprinkle with shredded mozzarella cheese. Fold the omelette in half and cook until cheese is melted.

Calories: 280

Lunch: Quinoa Salad with Chickpeas

Prep Time: 15 minutes

Ingredients:

1/2 cup cooked quinoa, 1/4 cup canned chickpeas, rinsed and drained

1/4 cup cucumber, diced, 1/4 cup cherry tomatoes, halved

1 tablespoon lemon juice, 1 tablespoon chopped fresh parsley

Instructions:

In a bowl, combine cooked quinoa, chickpeas, cucumber, and cherry tomatoes.

Drizzle with lemon juice and sprinkle with chopped parsley. Toss to combine.

Calories: 320

Dinner: Turkey Meatballs with Zucchini Noodles

Prep Time: 30 minutes

Ingredients:

4 oz ground turkey, 1/4 cup breadcrumbs (made from whole wheat bread)

1/4 cup grated Parmesan cheese, 1/2 teaspoon dried oregano

1/2 teaspoon garlic powder, Salt and pepper to taste

1 zucchini, spiralized into noodles, 1/2 cup marinara sauce (low-sodium)

Instructions:

Preheat oven to 375°F (190°C).

In a bowl, combine ground turkey, breadcrumbs, Parmesan cheese, dried oregano, garlic powder, salt, and pepper. Shape into meatballs.

Place meatballs on a baking sheet lined with parchment paper. Bake for 20-25 minutes or until cooked through.

In a skillet, heat marinara sauce over medium heat. Add zucchini noodles and cook until tender.

Serve turkey meatballs over zucchini noodles.

Calories: 380

Snack: Apple Slices with Almond Butter

Prep Time: 5 minutes

Ingredients:

1 medium apple, sliced

1 tablespoon almond butter

Instructions:

Arrange apple slices on a plate.

Serve with almond butter for dipping.

Calories: 150

Day 3:

Breakfast: Greek Yogurt Parfait

Prep Time: 5 minutes

Ingredients:

1/2 cup plain Greek yogurt

1/4 cup granola (low-sodium), 1/4 cup mixed berries

Instructions:

In a glass or bowl, layer Greek yogurt, granola, and mixed berries.

Repeat layers if desired.

Calories: 280

Lunch: Turkey and Avocado Wrap

Prep Time: 10 minutes

Ingredients:

2 oz sliced turkey breast, 1 small whole wheat tortilla

1/4 avocado, sliced, 1/4 cup spinach leaves, 1 tablespoon hummus

Instructions:

Lay the tortilla flat and spread hummus over it.

Layer with turkey slices, avocado slices, and spinach leaves.

Roll up the tortilla tightly.

Calories: 300

Dinner: Lentil Vegetable Soup

Prep Time: 30 minutes

Ingredients:

1/2 cup lentils, rinsed, 1 carrot, diced

1 celery stalk, diced, 1/4 onion, diced

2 cups low-sodium vegetable broth, 1 bay leaf

Salt and pepper to taste

Instructions:

In a pot, combine lentils, carrot, celery, onion, vegetable broth, and bay leaf.

Bring to a boil, then reduce heat and simmer for 20-25 minutes until lentils are tender.

Season with salt and pepper to taste before serving.

Calories: 350

Snack: Rice Cake with Cottage Cheese

Prep Time: 5 minutes

Ingredients:

1 rice cake

2 tablespoons low-fat cottage cheese

Instructions:

Spread cottage cheese over the rice cake.

Calories: 100

Day 4:

Breakfast: Spinach and Feta Breakfast Wrap

Prep Time: 10 minutes

Ingredients:

2 eggs, scrambled, 1 whole wheat tortilla

1/4 cup spinach leaves, 1 tablespoon crumbled feta cheese

Instructions:

Lay the tortilla flat and add scrambled eggs, spinach leaves, and feta cheese.

Roll up the tortilla and serve.

Calories: 290

Lunch: Tuna Salad Lettuce Wraps

Prep Time: 10 minutes

Ingredients:

1/2 can tuna, drained, 1 tablespoon Greek yogurt

1/4 cucumber, diced, 1 tablespoon chopped red onion

1 tablespoon chopped celery, Lettuce leaves for wrapping

Instructions:

In a bowl, mix tuna, Greek yogurt, cucumber, red onion, and celery.

Spoon the tuna salad onto lettuce leaves and wrap them up.

Calories: 280

Dinner: Baked Chicken with Roasted Vegetables

Prep Time: 40 minutes

Ingredients:

4 oz chicken breast, 1/2 cup bell peppers, sliced

1/2 cup zucchini, sliced, 1/4 onion, sliced

1 teaspoon olive oil, Salt and pepper to taste

Instructions:

Preheat oven to 375°F (190°C).

Place chicken breast on a baking sheet lined with parchment paper. Season with salt and pepper.

In a bowl, toss bell peppers, zucchini, and onion with olive oil, salt, and pepper. Spread them around the chicken on the baking sheet.

Bake for 25-30 minutes or until chicken is cooked through and vegetables are tender.

Calories: 350

Snack: Celery Sticks with Peanut Butter

Prep Time: 5 minutes

Ingredients:

2 celery sticks

2 tablespoons peanut butter (unsalted)

Instructions:

Spread peanut butter onto celery sticks.

Calories: 150

Day 5:

Breakfast: Chia Seed Pudding

Prep Time: 5 minutes (plus overnight chilling)

Ingredients:

2 tablespoons chia seeds, 1/2 cup almond milk (unsweetened)

1/4 teaspoon vanilla extract, 1/2 tablespoon honey (optional)

Instructions:

In a bowl, mix chia seeds, almond milk, vanilla extract, and honey (if using).

Cover and refrigerate overnight or for at least 2 hours until thickened.

Serve chilled.

Calories: 220

Lunch: Egg Salad Lettuce Wraps

Prep Time: 10 minutes

Ingredients:

2 hard-boiled eggs, chopped, 1 tablespoon Greek yogurt

1 teaspoon Dijon mustard, Salt and pepper to taste

Lettuce leaves for wrapping

Instructions:

In a bowl, mix chopped hard-boiled eggs, Greek yogurt, Dijon mustard, salt, and pepper.

Spoon the egg salad onto lettuce leaves and wrap them up.

Calories: 280

Dinner: Vegetable Stir-Fry with Brown Rice

Prep Time: 20 minutes

Ingredients:

1/2 cup mixed vegetables (such as bell peppers, broccoli, carrots), 2 oz tofu, cubed

1 teaspoon olive oil, 1 tablespoon low-sodium soy sauce, 1/2 cup cooked brown rice

Instructions:

Heat olive oil in a skillet over medium heat. Add tofu and cook until lightly browned.

Add mixed vegetables and stir-fry until tender.

Stir in cooked brown rice and soy sauce, cook for another 2-3 minutes.

Calories: 380

Snack: Cottage Cheese with Pineapple

Prep Time: 5 minutes

Ingredients:

1/2 cup low-fat cottage cheese

1/4 cup diced pineapple

Instructions:

Combine cottage cheese and diced pineapple in a bowl.

Calories: 150

Day 6:

Breakfast: Banana Almond Smoothie

Prep Time: 5 minutes

Ingredients:

1 ripe banana, 1 tablespoon almond butter

1/2 cup unsweetened almond milk, 1/4 teaspoon ground cinnamon

Instructions:

Place all ingredients in a blender.

Blend until smooth.

Serve immediately.

Calories: 280

Lunch: Quinoa and Black Bean Salad

Prep Time: 15 minutes

Ingredients:

1/2 cup cooked quinoa, 1/4 cup canned black beans, rinsed and drained

1/4 cup diced bell pepper, 1/4 cup diced cucumber

1 tablespoon chopped cilantro, 1 tablespoon lime juice

Instructions:

In a bowl, combine cooked quinoa, black beans, bell pepper, cucumber, cilantro, and lime juice.

Toss gently to combine.

Calories: 320

Dinner: Lemon Herb Baked Cod

Prep Time: 20 minutes

Ingredients:

4 oz cod fillet, 1 teaspoon olive oil

1/2 tablespoon fresh lemon juice, 1/2 teaspoon dried thyme

Salt and pepper to taste

Instructions:

Preheat oven to 375°F (190°C).

Place cod fillet on a baking sheet lined with parchment paper.

Drizzle with olive oil and lemon juice. Sprinkle with dried thyme, salt, and pepper.

Bake for 15-20 minutes or until fish flakes easily with a fork.

Calories: 300

Snack: Carrot Sticks with Hummus

Prep Time: 5 minutes

Ingredients:

1 medium carrot, cut into sticks

2 tablespoons hummus

Instructions:

Serve carrot sticks with hummus for dipping.

Calories: 100

Day 7:

Breakfast: Berry Protein Smoothie

Prep Time: 5 minutes

Ingredients:

1/2 cup mixed berries (such as strawberries, blueberries, raspberries), 1/2 cup unsweetened almond milk

1 scoop vanilla protein powder

Instructions:

Place all ingredients in a blender.

Blend until smooth.

Serve immediately.

Calories: 250

Lunch: Chickpea Salad

Prep Time: 10 minutes

Ingredients:

1/2 cup canned chickpeas, rinsed and drained, 1/4 cup diced cucumber

1/4 cup diced tomato, 1/4 cup diced red onion

1 tablespoon chopped fresh parsley, 1 tablespoon olive oil, 1 tablespoon lemon juice

Instructions:

In a bowl, combine chickpeas, cucumber, tomato, red onion, and parsley.

Drizzle with olive oil and lemon juice. Toss to combine.

Calories: 320

Dinner: Vegetable and Lentil Curry

Prep Time: 30 minutes

Ingredients:

1/2 cup cooked lentils, 1/2 cup diced eggplant

1/2 cup diced zucchini, 1/4 cup diced onion

1/4 cup diced bell pepper, 1/2 cup canned diced tomatoes

1/2 cup low-sodium vegetable broth, 1 teaspoon curry powder, Salt and pepper to taste

Instructions:

In a skillet, sauté onion and bell pepper until softened.

Add diced eggplant, zucchini, canned tomatoes, vegetable broth, curry powder, salt, and pepper. Cook until vegetables are tender.

Stir in cooked lentils and cook for another 5 minutes.

Serve hot.

Calories: 350

Snack: Rice Cake with Avocado
Prep Time: 5 minutes
Ingredients:
1 rice cake
1/4 avocado, mashed

Instructions:
Spread mashed avocado onto the rice cake.
Calories: 150

Day 8:

Breakfast: Berry Chia Pudding
Prep Time: 5 minutes (plus overnight chilling)
Ingredients:
2 tablespoons chia seeds, 1/2 cup unsweetened almond milk
1/4 teaspoon vanilla extract, 1/2 cup mixed berries

Instructions:

In a bowl, mix chia seeds, almond milk, and vanilla extract.

Cover and refrigerate overnight or for at least 2 hours until thickened.

Serve chilled, topped with mixed berries.

Calories: 230

Lunch: Mediterranean Chickpea Salad

Prep Time: 15 minutes

Ingredients:

1/2 cup canned chickpeas, rinsed and drained, 1/4 cup diced cucumber

1/4 cup diced tomato, 1/4 cup diced red bell pepper, 1 tablespoon chopped fresh parsley

1 tablespoon olive oil, 1 tablespoon lemon juice, 1 tablespoon crumbled feta cheese

Instructions:

In a bowl, combine chickpeas, cucumber, tomato, red bell pepper, and parsley.

Drizzle with olive oil and lemon juice. Toss to combine.

Sprinkle with crumbled feta cheese before serving.

Calories: 320

Dinner: Grilled Lemon Herb Chicken

Prep Time: 25 minutes

Ingredients:

4 oz chicken breast, 1 tablespoon olive oil. 1 tablespoon lemon juice

1/2 teaspoon dried oregano, Salt and pepper to taste

Instructions:

In a bowl, mix olive oil, lemon juice, dried oregano, salt, and pepper.

Marinate chicken breast in the mixture for 15-20 minutes.

Heat a grill pan over medium-high heat. Grill chicken for 6-8 minutes on each side or until cooked through.

Calories: 320

Snack: Celery Sticks with Cream Cheese

Prep Time: 5 minutes

Ingredients:

2 celery sticks

2 tablespoons cream cheese (low-fat)

Instructions:

Spread cream cheese onto celery sticks.

Calories: 120

Day 9:

Breakfast: Veggie Egg Muffins

Prep Time: 20 minutes

Ingredients:

2 eggs, 1/4 cup diced bell pepper

1/4 cup diced onion, 1/4 cup chopped spinach, Salt and pepper to taste

Instructions:

Preheat oven to 350°F (175°C). Grease muffin tin or line with paper liners.

In a bowl, beat eggs and season with salt and pepper.

Stir in diced bell pepper, onion, and chopped spinach.

Pour egg mixture into muffin cups, filling each about 3/4 full.

Bake for 15-20 minutes or until eggs are set.

Calories: 180

Lunch: Lentil and Vegetable Stir-Fry

Prep Time: 20 minutes

Ingredients:

1/2 cup cooked lentils, 1/2 cup mixed vegetables (such as bell peppers, broccoli, carrots)

1 tablespoon low-sodium soy sauce, 1 teaspoon sesame oil

Instructions:

Heat sesame oil in a skillet over medium heat.

Add mixed vegetables and stir-fry until tender.

Stir in cooked lentils and soy sauce, cook for another 2-3 minutes.

Calories: 290

Dinner: Baked Cod with Asparagus

Prep Time: 25 minutes

Ingredients:

4 oz cod fillet. 1/2 bunch asparagus, trimmed

1 tablespoon olive oil, 1/2 tablespoon lemon juice, Salt and pepper to taste

Instructions:

Preheat oven to 375°F (190°C).

Place cod fillet on a baking sheet lined with parchment paper.

Arrange asparagus around the cod. Drizzle with olive oil and lemon juice. Season with salt and pepper.

Bake for 15-20 minutes or until fish flakes easily with a fork.

Calories: 320

Snack: Apple Slices with Peanut Butter

Prep Time: 5 minutes

Ingredients:

1 medium apple, sliced, 2 tablespoons peanut butter (unsalted)

Instructions:

Serve apple slices with peanut butter for dipping.

Calories: 200

Day 10:

Breakfast: Greek Yogurt with Granola

Prep Time: 5 minutes

Ingredients:

1/2 cup plain Greek yogurt

1/4 cup granola (low-sodium)

1/4 cup mixed berries

Instructions:

In a bowl, layer Greek yogurt, granola, and mixed berries.

Repeat layers if desired.

Calories: 280

Lunch: Turkey and Avocado Wrap

Prep Time: 10 minutes

Ingredients:

2 oz sliced turkey breast, 1 small whole wheat tortilla

1/4 avocado, sliced, 1/4 cup spinach leaves, 1 tablespoon hummus

Instructions:

Lay the tortilla flat and spread hummus over it.

Layer with turkey slices, avocado slices, and spinach leaves.

Roll up the tortilla tightly.

Calories: 300

Dinner: Lentil Vegetable Soup

Prep Time: 30 minutes

Ingredients:

1/2 cup lentils, rinsed, 1 carrot, diced

1 celery stalk, diced, 1/4 onion, diced

2 cups low-sodium vegetable broth

1 bay leaf, Salt and pepper to taste

Instructions:

In a pot, combine lentils, carrot, celery, onion, vegetable broth, and bay leaf.

Bring to a boil, then reduce heat and simmer for 20-25 minutes until lentils are tender.

Season with salt and pepper to taste before serving.

Calories: 350

Snack: Rice Cake with Cottage Cheese

Prep Time: 5 minutes

Ingredients:

1 rice cake

2 tablespoons low-fat cottage cheese

Instructions:

Spread cottage cheese over the rice cake.

Calories: 100

Day 11:

Breakfast: Spinach and Feta Breakfast Wrap

Prep Time: 10 minutes

Ingredients:

2 eggs, scrambled, 1 whole wheat tortilla

1/4 cup spinach leaves, 1 tablespoon crumbled feta cheese

Instructions:

Lay the tortilla flat and add scrambled eggs, spinach leaves, and feta cheese.

Roll up the tortilla and serve.

Calories: 290

Lunch: Tuna Salad Lettuce Wraps

Prep Time: 10 minutes

Ingredients:

1/2 can tuna, drained, 1 tablespoon Greek yogurt

1 teaspoon Dijon mustard, Salt and pepper to taste

Lettuce leaves for wrapping

Instructions:

In a bowl, mix tuna, Greek yogurt, Dijon mustard, salt, and pepper.

Spoon the tuna salad onto lettuce leaves and wrap them up.

Calories: 280

Dinner: Vegetable Stir-Fry with Brown Rice

Prep Time: 20 minutes

Ingredients:

1/2 cup mixed vegetables (such as bell peppers, broccoli, carrots), 2 oz tofu, cubed

1 teaspoon olive oil, 1 tablespoon low-sodium soy sauce

1/2 cup cooked brown rice

Instructions:

Heat olive oil in a skillet over medium heat. Add tofu and cook until lightly browned.

Add mixed vegetables and stir-fry until tender.

Stir in cooked brown rice and soy sauce, cook for another 2-3 minutes.

Serve hot.

Calories: 380

Snack: Celery Sticks with Peanut Butter

Prep Time: 5 minutes

Ingredients:

2 celery sticks

2 tablespoons peanut butter (unsalted)

Instructions:

Spread peanut butter onto celery sticks.

Calories: 150

Day 12:

Breakfast: Chia Seed Pudding

Prep Time: 5 minutes (plus overnight chilling)

Ingredients:

2 tablespoons chia seeds

1/2 cup almond milk (unsweetened)

1/4 teaspoon vanilla extract

1/2 tablespoon honey (optional)

Instructions:

In a bowl, mix chia seeds, almond milk, vanilla extract, and honey (if using).

Cover and refrigerate overnight or for at least 2 hours until thickened.

Serve chilled.

Calories: 220

Lunch: Egg Salad Lettuce Wraps

Prep Time: 10 minutes

Ingredients:

2 hard-boiled eggs, chopped, 1 tablespoon Greek yogurt

1 teaspoon Dijon mustard, Salt and pepper to taste

Lettuce leaves for wrapping

Instructions:

In a bowl, mix chopped hard-boiled eggs, Greek yogurt, Dijon mustard, salt, and pepper.

Spoon the egg salad onto lettuce leaves and wrap them up.

Calories: 280

Dinner: Vegetable and Lentil Curry

Prep Time: 30 minutes

Ingredients:

1/2 cup cooked lentils, 1/2 cup diced eggplant

1/2 cup diced zucchini, 1/4 cup diced onion

1/4 cup diced bell pepper, 1/2 cup canned diced tomatoes

1/2 cup low-sodium vegetable broth, 1 teaspoon curry powder, Salt and pepper to taste

Instructions:

In a skillet, sauté onion and bell pepper until softened.

Add diced eggplant, zucchini, canned tomatoes, vegetable broth, curry powder, salt, and pepper. Cook until vegetables are tender.

Stir in cooked lentils and cook for another 5 minutes.

Serve hot.

Calories: 350

Snack: Rice Cake with Avocado

Prep Time: 5 minutes

Ingredients:

1 rice cake

1/4 avocado, mashed

Instructions:

Spread mashed avocado onto the rice cake.

Calories: 150

Day 13:

Breakfast: Berry Protein Smoothie

Prep Time: 5 minutes

Ingredients:

1/2 cup mixed berries (such as strawberries, blueberries, raspberries)

1/2 cup unsweetened almond milk

1 scoop vanilla protein powder

Instructions:

Place all ingredients in a blender.

Blend until smooth.

Serve immediately.

Calories: 250

Lunch: Chickpea Salad

Prep Time: 10 minutes

Ingredients:

1/2 cup canned chickpeas, rinsed and drained, 1/4 cup diced cucumber

1/4 cup diced tomato, 1/4 cup diced red onion

1 tablespoon chopped fresh parsley, 1 tablespoon olive oil, 1 tablespoon lemon juice

Instructions:

In a bowl, combine chickpeas, cucumber, tomato, red onion, and parsley.

Drizzle with olive oil and lemon juice. Toss to combine.

Calories: 320

Dinner: Lemon Herb Baked Cod

Prep Time: 20 minutes

Ingredients:

4 oz cod fillet, 1 teaspoon olive oil

1/2 tablespoon fresh lemon juice, 1/2 teaspoon dried thyme, Salt and pepper to taste

Instructions:

Preheat oven to 375°F (190°C).

Place cod fillet on a baking sheet lined with parchment paper.

Drizzle with olive oil and lemon juice. Sprinkle with dried thyme, salt, and pepper.

Bake for 15-20 minutes or until fish flakes easily with a fork.

Calories: 320

Snack: Carrot Sticks with Hummus

Prep Time: 5 minutes

Ingredients:

1 medium carrot, cut into sticks

2 tablespoons hummus

Instructions:

Serve carrot sticks with hummus for dipping.

Calories: 100

Day 14:

Breakfast: Banana Almond Smoothie

Prep Time: 5 minutes

Ingredients:

1 ripe banana, 1 tablespoon almond butter

1/2 cup unsweetened almond milk, 1/4 teaspoon ground cinnamon

Instructions:

Place all ingredients in a blender.

Blend until smooth.

Serve immediately.

Calories: 280

Lunch: Quinoa and Black Bean Salad

Prep Time: 15 minutes

Ingredients:

1/2 cup cooked quinoa, 1/4 cup canned black beans, rinsed and drained

1/4 cup diced bell pepper, 1/4 cup diced cucumber

1 tablespoon chopped cilantro, 1 tablespoon lime juice

Instructions:

In a bowl, combine cooked quinoa, black beans, bell pepper, cucumber, cilantro, and lime juice.

Toss gently to combine.

Calories: 320

Dinner: Vegetable and Lentil Soup

Prep Time: 30 minutes

Ingredients:

1/2 cup cooked lentils, 1 carrot, diced

1 celery stalk, diced, 1/4 onion, diced

2 cups low-sodium vegetable broth, 1 bay leaf, Salt and pepper to taste

Instructions:

In a pot, combine lentils, carrot, celery, onion, vegetable broth, and bay leaf.

Bring to a boil, then reduce heat and simmer for 20-25 minutes until vegetables are tender.

Season with salt and pepper to taste before serving.

Calories: 350

Snack: Rice Cake with Peanut Butter
Prep Time: 5 minutes
Ingredients:
1 rice cake
2 tablespoons peanut butter (unsalted)
Instructions:
Spread peanut butter onto the rice cake.
Calories: 200

Day 15:

Breakfast: Spinach and Mushroom Omelette
Prep Time: 10 minutes
Ingredients:
2 eggs, 1/4 cup chopped spinach
1/4 cup sliced mushrooms, 1 tablespoon diced onion, Salt and pepper to taste

Instructions:
In a bowl, beat eggs and season with salt and pepper.

Heat a non-stick skillet over medium heat and add chopped spinach, sliced mushrooms, and diced onion.

Pour beaten eggs over the vegetables and cook until the omelette is set.

Fold the omelette in half and serve hot.

Calories: 250

Lunch: Quinoa Salad with Lemon Herb Dressing

Prep Time: 15 minutes

Ingredients:

1/2 cup cooked quinoa, 1/4 cup diced cucumber

1/4 cup diced tomato, 1/4 cup diced bell pepper

1 tablespoon chopped parsley, 1 tablespoon lemon juice, 1/2 tablespoon olive oil

Instructions:

In a bowl, combine cooked quinoa, diced cucumber, tomato, bell pepper, and parsley.

In a small bowl, whisk together lemon juice and olive oil to make the dressing.

Drizzle the dressing over the quinoa salad and toss to combine.

Calories: 280

Dinner: Baked Salmon with Steamed Broccoli

Prep Time: 20 minutes

Ingredients:

4 oz salmon fillet, 1/2 tablespoon olive oil

1/2 tablespoon lemon juice, 1/4 teaspoon dried dill

Salt and pepper to taste, 1 cup broccoli florets

Instructions:

Preheat oven to 375°F (190°C).

Place salmon fillet on a baking sheet lined with parchment paper.

Drizzle with olive oil and lemon juice. Sprinkle with dried dill, salt, and pepper.

Bake for 15-20 minutes or until salmon is cooked through.

Steam broccoli florets until tender.

Calories: 350

Snack: Greek Yogurt with Berries

Prep Time: 5 minutes

Ingredients:

1/2 cup plain Greek yogurt

1/4 cup mixed berries

Instructions:

In a bowl, layer Greek yogurt and mixed berries.

Calories: 150

Day 16:

Breakfast: Avocado Toast

Prep Time: 5 minutes

Ingredients:

1 slice whole grain bread, toasted

1/4 avocado, mashed

Pinch of red pepper flakes

Instructions:

Spread mashed avocado on top of toasted bread.

Sprinkle with red pepper flakes.

Calories: 200

Lunch: Chicken and Vegetable Stir-Fry

Prep Time: 20 minutes

Ingredients:

4 oz chicken breast, sliced

1/2 cup mixed vegetables (such as bell peppers, broccoli, carrots)

1 tablespoon low-sodium soy sauce

1 teaspoon sesame oil

Instructions:

Heat sesame oil in a skillet over medium heat.

Add sliced chicken breast and cook until browned and cooked through.

Add mixed vegetables and stir-fry until tender.

Stir in low-sodium soy sauce and cook for another 2-3 minutes.

Calories: 320

Dinner: Turkey Meatballs with Zucchini Noodles

Prep Time: 30 minutes

Ingredients:

4 oz ground turkey

1/4 cup whole wheat breadcrumbs, 1 egg

1/2 teaspoon garlic powder, 1/4 teaspoon dried oregano

Salt and pepper to taste, 1 medium zucchini, spiralized, 1/4 cup marinara sauce (low-sodium)

Instructions:

Preheat oven to 375°F (190°C).

In a bowl, combine ground turkey, breadcrumbs, egg, garlic powder, dried oregano, salt, and pepper. Mix well.

Shape the mixture into meatballs and place them on a baking sheet lined with parchment paper.

Bake for 20-25 minutes or until meatballs are cooked through.

In a separate skillet, sauté spiralized zucchini until tender. Serve with turkey meatballs and marinara sauce.

Calories: 350

Snack: Cottage Cheese with Pineapple

Prep Time: 5 minutes

Ingredients:

1/2 cup low-fat cottage cheese

1/4 cup diced pineapple

Instructions:

In a bowl, combine cottage cheese and diced pineapple.

Calories: 150

Day 17:

Breakfast: Blueberry Oatmeal

Prep Time: 10 minutes

Ingredients:

1/2 cup rolled oats, 1 cup water

1/4 cup fresh blueberries, 1 tablespoon chopped almonds

Instructions:

In a saucepan, bring water to a boil. Stir in rolled oats and reduce heat to low. Cook for 5 minutes, stirring occasionally.

Remove from heat and let it sit for 2-3 minutes.

Top with fresh blueberries, chopped almonds, and honey (if using).

Calories: 250

Lunch: Caprese Salad

Prep Time: 10 minutes

Ingredients:

1 medium tomato, sliced

1/4 cup fresh mozzarella cheese, sliced

2 fresh basil leaves

1/2 tablespoon balsamic glaze

Instructions:

Arrange tomato and mozzarella slices on a plate.

Top with fresh basil leaves and drizzle with balsamic glaze.

Calories: 280

Dinner: Vegetable and Lentil Curry

Prep Time: 30 minutes

Ingredients:

1/2 cup cooked lentils, 1/2 cup diced eggplant

1/2 cup diced zucchini, 1/4 cup diced onion

1/4 cup diced bell pepper, 1/2 cup canned diced tomatoes

1/2 cup low-sodium vegetable broth, 1 teaspoon curry powder, Salt and pepper to taste

Instructions:

In a skillet, sauté onion and bell pepper until softened.

Add diced eggplant, zucchini, canned tomatoes, vegetable broth, curry powder, salt, and pepper. Cook until vegetables are tender.

Stir in cooked lentils and cook for another 5 minutes.

Serve hot.

Calories: 350

Snack: Apple Slices with Almond Butter

Prep Time: 5 minutes

Ingredients:

1 medium apple, sliced

2 tablespoons almond butter (unsalted)

Instructions:

Serve apple slices with almond butter for dipping.

Calories: 200

Day 18:

Breakfast: Greek Yogurt Parfait

Prep Time: 5 minutes

Ingredients:

1/2 cup plain Greek yogurt

1/4 cup granola (low-sugar)

1/4 cup mixed berries

Instructions:

In a glass, layer Greek yogurt, granola, and mixed berries.

Calories: 280

Lunch: Turkey and Avocado Wrap

Prep Time: 10 minutes

Ingredients:

2 oz sliced turkey breast, 1 whole wheat tortilla

1/4 avocado, sliced, 1/4 cup shredded lettuce

Instructions:

Lay the tortilla flat and add sliced turkey breast, avocado slices, and shredded lettuce.

Roll up the tortilla and serve.

Calories: 320

Dinner: Grilled Chicken with Roasted Vegetables

Prep Time: 30 minutes

Ingredients:

4 oz chicken breast

1/2 cup mixed vegetables (such as bell peppers, zucchini, cherry tomatoes), 1 teaspoon olive oil, 1/2 teaspoon dried herbs (such as thyme, rosemary, oregano)

Salt and pepper to taste

Instructions:

Preheat grill to medium-high heat.

Brush chicken breast and mixed vegetables with olive oil and season with dried herbs, salt, and pepper.

Grill chicken for 6-8 minutes per side or until cooked through, and grill vegetables until tender.

Calories: 350

Snack: Cucumber Slices with Hummus

Prep Time: 5 minutes

Ingredients:

1 medium cucumber, sliced

2 tablespoons hummus

Instructions:

Serve cucumber slices with hummus for dipping.

Calories: 100

Day 19:

Breakfast: Berry Smoothie Bowl

Prep Time: 5 minutes

Ingredients:

1/2 cup mixed berries (such as strawberries, blueberries, raspberries)

1/2 cup plain Greek yogurt

1/4 cup granola (low-sugar)

Instructions:

In a bowl, layer mixed berries and Greek yogurt.

Top with granola.

Calories: 250

Lunch: Chicken Caesar Salad

Prep Time: 15 minutes

Ingredients:

2 oz grilled chicken breast, sliced

2 cups chopped romaine lettuce, 1/4 cup cherry tomatoes, halved

1 tablespoon grated Parmesan cheese, 1 tablespoon Caesar dressing (low-sodium)

Instructions:

In a bowl, combine grilled chicken breast, chopped romaine lettuce, cherry tomatoes, and grated Parmesan cheese.

Drizzle with Caesar dressing and toss to combine.

Calories: 280

Dinner: Baked Cod with Lemon Garlic Sauce

Prep Time: 25 minutes

Ingredients:

4 oz cod fillet, 1 teaspoon olive oil

1/2 tablespoon lemon juice, 1/2 teaspoon minced garlic, Salt and pepper to taste

Instructions:

Preheat oven to 375°F (190°C).

Place cod fillet on a baking sheet lined with parchment paper.

Drizzle with olive oil and lemon juice. Sprinkle with minced garlic, salt, and pepper.

Bake for 15-20 minutes or until fish flakes easily with a fork.

Calories: 300

Snack: Mixed Nuts

Prep Time: 5 minutes

Ingredients:

1/4 cup mixed nuts (such as almonds, walnuts, cashews)

Instructions:

Enjoy a handful of mixed nuts as a snack.

Calories: 200

Day 20:

Breakfast: Veggie Egg Muffins

Prep Time: 20 minutes

Ingredients:

2 eggs, 1/4 cup diced bell pepper

1/4 cup diced onion, 1/4 cup diced tomato

1/4 cup chopped spinach, Salt and pepper to taste

Instructions:

Preheat oven to 350°F (175°C) and grease a muffin tin.

In a bowl, whisk eggs and season with salt and pepper.

Stir in diced bell pepper, onion, tomato, and chopped spinach.

Pour the mixture into the muffin tin, filling each cup about 3/4 full.

Bake for 15-20 minutes or until the egg muffins are set.

Calories: 200

Lunch: Turkey and Vegetable Wrap

Prep Time: 10 minutes

Ingredients:

2 oz sliced turkey breast, 1 whole wheat tortilla

1/4 cup sliced cucumber, 1/4 cup shredded lettuce

Instructions:

Lay the tortilla flat and add sliced turkey breast, sliced cucumber, and shredded lettuce.

Roll up the tortilla and serve.

Calories: 280

Dinner: Lemon Herb Grilled Chicken

Prep Time: 25 minutes

Ingredients:

4 oz chicken breast, 1 teaspoon olive oil

1/2 tablespoon lemon juice, 1/2 teaspoon dried herbs (such as thyme, rosemary, oregano)

Salt and pepper to taste

Instructions:

In a bowl, whisk together olive oil, lemon juice, dried herbs, salt, and pepper.

Marinate chicken breast in the mixture for 15 minutes.

Preheat grill to medium-high heat and grill chicken for 6-8 minutes per side or until cooked through.

Calories: 320

Snack: Rice Cake with Cottage Cheese

Prep Time: 5 minutes

Ingredients:

1 rice cake, 2 tablespoons low-fat cottage cheese

Instructions:

Spread cottage cheese onto the rice cake.

Calories: 150

Day 21:

Breakfast: Banana Chia Seed Pudding

Prep Time: 5 minutes (+ overnight chilling)

Ingredients:

1 ripe banana, mashed, 1/4 cup chia seeds

1/2 cup unsweetened almond milk, 1/4 teaspoon vanilla extract

Instructions:

In a bowl, mix mashed banana, chia seeds, almond milk, and vanilla extract.

Refrigerate overnight or for at least 4 hours until the mixture thickens.

Serve chilled.

Calories: 230

Lunch: Lentil Salad with Feta

Prep Time: 15 minutes

Ingredients:

1/2 cup cooked lentils, 1/4 cup diced cucumber

1/4 cup diced bell pepper, 2 tablespoons crumbled feta cheese

1 tablespoon chopped parsley, 1 tablespoon balsamic vinegar

Instructions:

In a bowl, combine cooked lentils, diced cucumber, diced bell pepper, crumbled feta cheese, chopped parsley, and balsamic vinegar.

Toss gently to combine.

Calories: 300

Dinner: Grilled Vegetable Quinoa Bowl

Prep Time: 30 minutes

Ingredients:

1/2 cup cooked quinoa, 1/2 cup mixed grilled vegetables (such as zucchini, bell peppers, eggplant)

2 tablespoons crumbled goat cheese, 1 tablespoon chopped fresh basil, 1 tablespoon balsamic glaze

Instructions:

In a bowl, layer cooked quinoa, mixed grilled vegetables, crumbled goat cheese, and chopped fresh basil.

Drizzle with balsamic glaze before serving.

Calories: 350

Snack: Edamame

Prep Time: 5 minutes

Ingredients:

1/2 cup cooked edamame (shelled)

Instructions:

Enjoy cooked edamame as a nutritious snack.

Calories: 100

Day 22:

Breakfast: Berry Smoothie

Prep Time: 5 minutes

Ingredients:

1/2 cup mixed berries (such as strawberries, blueberries, raspberries), 1/2 cup unsweetened almond milk

1/2 banana, 1 tablespoon chia seeds

Instructions:

Blend mixed berries, almond milk, banana, and chia seeds until smooth.

Serve immediately.

Calories: 200

Lunch: Tuna Salad Wrap

Prep Time: 10 minutes

Ingredients:

2 oz canned tuna, drained, 1 tablespoon Greek yogurt

1/4 cup diced cucumber, 1/4 cup diced bell pepper, 1 whole wheat tortilla

Instructions:

In a bowl, mix canned tuna, Greek yogurt, diced cucumber, and diced bell pepper.

Lay the tortilla flat and spread the tuna salad mixture evenly.

Roll up the tortilla and serve.

Calories: 280

Dinner: Lemon Garlic Shrimp with Brown Rice

Prep Time: 25 minutes

Ingredients:

4 oz shrimp, peeled and deveined, 1 teaspoon olive oil

1/2 tablespoon lemon juice, 1/2 teaspoon minced garlic

Salt and pepper to taste, 1/2 cup cooked brown rice

Instructions:

In a bowl, toss shrimp with olive oil, lemon juice, minced garlic, salt, and pepper.

Heat a skillet over medium heat and cook shrimp for 2-3 minutes on each side until pink and cooked through.

Serve shrimp over cooked brown rice.

Calories: 320

Snack: Carrot Sticks with Hummus

Prep Time: 5 minutes

Ingredients:

1 medium carrot, cut into sticks

2 tablespoons hummus

Instructions:

Enjoy carrot sticks with hummus as a healthy snack.

Calories: 100

Day 23:

Breakfast: Greek Yogurt with Almonds and Honey

Prep Time: 5 minutes

Ingredients:

1/2 cup plain Greek yogurt

1 tablespoon sliced almonds

1 teaspoon honey

Instructions:

In a bowl, top Greek yogurt with sliced almonds and drizzle with honey.

Calories: 220

Lunch: Chicken Caesar Wrap

Prep Time: 10 minutes

Ingredients:

2 oz grilled chicken breast, sliced

1 whole wheat tortilla

1/2 cup chopped romaine lettuce

1 tablespoon grated Parmesan cheese

1 tablespoon Caesar dressing (low-sodium)

Instructions:

Lay the tortilla flat and add sliced grilled chicken breast, chopped romaine lettuce, grated Parmesan cheese, and Caesar dressing.

Roll up the tortilla and serve.

Calories: 320

Dinner: Baked Salmon with Asparagus

Prep Time: 25 minutes

Ingredients:

4 oz salmon fillet, 1/2 tablespoon olive oil

1/2 tablespoon lemon juice, Salt and pepper to taste

1/2 bunch asparagus, trimmed

Instructions:

Preheat oven to 375°F (190°C).

Place salmon fillet on a baking sheet lined with parchment paper.

Drizzle with olive oil and lemon juice. Season with salt and pepper.

Arrange asparagus around the salmon.

Bake for 15-20 minutes or until salmon is cooked through and asparagus is tender.

Calories: 350

Snack: Rice Cake with Peanut Butter

Prep Time: 5 minutes

Ingredients:

1 rice cake

1 tablespoon peanut butter (unsalted)

Instructions:

Spread peanut butter onto the rice cake.

Calories: 200

Day 24:

Breakfast: Veggie Scramble

Prep Time: 10 minutes

Ingredients:

2 eggs

1/4 cup diced bell pepper, 1/4 cup diced onion

1/4 cup diced tomato, Salt and pepper to taste

Instructions:

In a skillet, sauté diced bell pepper and onion until softened.

Add diced tomato and cook for another 2 minutes.

Beat eggs in a bowl and pour into the skillet with the vegetables.

Cook, stirring occasionally, until eggs are scrambled and cooked through.

Season with salt and pepper to taste.

Calories: 250

Lunch: Quinoa Salad with Chickpeas

Prep Time: 15 minutes

Ingredients:

1/2 cup cooked quinoa, 1/4 cup cooked chickpeas

1/4 cup diced cucumber, 1/4 cup diced bell pepper

1 tablespoon chopped parsley, 1 tablespoon lemon juice

1/2 tablespoon olive oil

Instructions:

In a bowl, combine cooked quinoa, cooked chickpeas, diced cucumber, diced bell pepper, and chopped parsley.

In a small bowl, whisk together lemon juice and olive oil to make the dressing.

Drizzle the dressing over the quinoa salad and toss to combine.

Calories: 280

Dinner: Turkey Meatloaf with Mashed Cauliflower

Prep Time: 40 minutes

Ingredients:

4 oz ground turkey, 1/4 cup rolled oats

1/4 cup diced onion, 1/4 cup diced bell pepper

1/4 cup marinara sauce (low-sodium), 1/2 head cauliflower, chopped

1/4 cup low-fat milk, Salt and pepper to taste

Instructions:

Preheat oven to 375°F (190°C).

In a bowl, combine ground turkey, rolled oats, diced onion, diced bell pepper, and marinara sauce. Mix well.

Transfer the mixture to a loaf pan and bake for 30 minutes.

Meanwhile, steam cauliflower until tender. Drain and mash with a potato masher.

Stir in low-fat milk and season with salt and pepper.

Serve turkey meatloaf with mashed cauliflower.

Calories: 350

Snack: Greek Yogurt with Berries

Prep Time: 5 minutes

Ingredients:

1/2 cup plain Greek yogurt

1/4 cup mixed berries

Instructions:

Top Greek yogurt with mixed berries.

Calories: 150

Day 25:

Breakfast: Spinach and Feta Omelette

Prep Time: 10 minutes

Ingredients:

2 eggs

1/4 cup chopped spinach

1 tablespoon crumbled feta cheese

Salt and pepper to taste

Instructions:

In a bowl, beat eggs and season with salt and pepper.

Heat a non-stick skillet over medium heat and pour in the beaten eggs.

Sprinkle chopped spinach and crumbled feta cheese over one half of the omelette.

Fold the other half of the omelette over the filling and cook for another 2 minutes until the cheese is melted.

Serve hot.

Calories: 250

Lunch: Turkey and Vegetable Stir-Fry

Prep Time: 15 minutes

Ingredients:

2 oz sliced turkey breast

1/2 cup mixed vegetables (such as bell peppers, broccoli, snap peas)

1 tablespoon low-sodium soy sauce

1/2 tablespoon sesame oil

1/2 teaspoon minced garlic

1/2 teaspoon grated ginger

Instructions:

Heat sesame oil in a skillet over medium-high heat.

Add sliced turkey breast and cook until browned.

Add mixed vegetables, minced garlic, and grated ginger. Stir-fry for 3-4 minutes until vegetables are tender-crisp.

Stir in low-sodium soy sauce and cook for another minute.

Serve hot.

Calories: 300

Dinner: Stuffed Bell Peppers

Prep Time: 40 minutes

Ingredients:

2 bell peppers, halved and seeds removed

4 oz lean ground beef, 1/4 cup cooked quinoa

1/4 cup diced tomatoes, 1/4 cup diced onion

1/4 cup diced zucchini, 1/4 cup shredded mozzarella cheese

1/2 teaspoon dried herbs (such as oregano, basil), Salt and pepper to taste

Instructions:

Preheat oven to 375°F (190°C).

In a skillet, cook lean ground beef until browned. Drain excess fat.

In a bowl, mix cooked ground beef, cooked quinoa, diced tomatoes, diced onion, diced zucchini, shredded mozzarella cheese, dried herbs, salt, and pepper.

Stuff the halved bell peppers with the mixture.

Place stuffed bell peppers in a baking dish and bake for 25-30 minutes until peppers are tender.

Calories: 350

Snack: Cottage Cheese with Pineapple

Prep Time: 5 minutes

Ingredients:

1/2 cup low-fat cottage cheese

1/4 cup diced pineapple

Instructions:

Top cottage cheese with diced pineapple.

Calories: 150

Day 26:

Breakfast: Avocado Toast

Prep Time: 5 minutes

Ingredients:

1 slice whole grain bread, toasted

1/4 avocado, mashed

Pinch of red pepper flakes

Instructions:

Spread mashed avocado on toasted whole grain bread.

Sprinkle with red pepper flakes.

Calories: 200

Lunch: Chickpea Salad

Prep Time: 15 minutes

Ingredients:

1/2 cup cooked chickpeas

1/4 cup diced cucumber, 1/4 cup diced bell pepper

1/4 cup diced tomato, 1 tablespoon chopped parsley

1 tablespoon lemon juice, 1/2 tablespoon olive oil

Instructions:

In a bowl, combine cooked chickpeas, diced cucumber, diced bell pepper, diced tomato, chopped parsley, lemon juice, and olive oil.

Toss gently to combine.

Calories: 280

Dinner: Baked Chicken with Roasted Vegetables

Prep Time: 40 minutes

Ingredients:

4 oz chicken breast

1 teaspoon olive oil

1/2 cup mixed vegetables (such as carrots, broccoli, cauliflower)

1/2 teaspoon dried herbs (such as thyme, rosemary, oregano)

Salt and pepper to taste

Instructions:

Preheat oven to 375°F (190°C).

Place chicken breast on a baking sheet lined with parchment paper.

Drizzle with olive oil and season with dried herbs, salt, and pepper.

Arrange mixed vegetables around the chicken.

Bake for 25-30 minutes or until chicken is cooked through and vegetables are tender.

Calories: 350

Snack: Rice Cake with Avocado

Prep Time: 5 minutes

Ingredients:

1 rice cake

1/4 avocado, sliced

Instructions:

Top rice cake with sliced avocado.

Calories: 150

Day 27:

Breakfast: Cottage Cheese and Pineapple Bowl

Prep Time: 5 minutes

Ingredients:

1/2 cup low-fat cottage cheese

1/4 cup diced pineapple

Instructions:

In a bowl, combine low-fat cottage cheese and diced pineapple.

Calories: 150

Lunch: Quinoa Stuffed Bell Peppers

Prep Time: 40 minutes

Ingredients:

2 bell peppers, halved and seeds removed

1/2 cup cooked quinoa

1/4 cup black beans, drained and rinsed

1/4 cup diced tomatoes

1/4 cup diced onion

1/4 cup shredded cheddar cheese

1/2 teaspoon chili powder

Salt and pepper to taste

Instructions:

Preheat oven to 375°F (190°C).

In a bowl, mix cooked quinoa, black beans, diced tomatoes, diced onion, shredded cheddar cheese, chili powder, salt, and pepper.

Stuff the halved bell peppers with the quinoa mixture.

Place stuffed bell peppers in a baking dish and bake for 25-30 minutes until peppers are tender and filling is heated through.

Calories: 350

Dinner: Lemon Herb Tilapia with Steamed Broccoli

Prep Time: 20 minutes

Ingredients:

4 oz tilapia fillet

1/2 tablespoon olive oil

1/2 tablespoon lemon juice

1/2 teaspoon dried herbs (such as parsley, dill, thyme)

Salt and pepper to taste

1 cup steamed broccoli florets

Instructions:

Preheat oven to 375°F (190°C).

Place tilapia fillet on a baking sheet lined with parchment paper.

Drizzle with olive oil and lemon juice. Sprinkle with dried herbs, salt, and pepper.

Bake for 12-15 minutes or until fish is cooked through and flakes easily with a fork.

Serve with steamed broccoli on the side.

Calories: 300

Snack: Apple Slices with Almond Butter

Prep Time: 5 minutes

Ingredients:

1 medium apple, sliced

1 tablespoon almond butter

Instructions:

Dip apple slices in almond butter.

Calories: 200

Day 28:

Breakfast: Spinach and Mushroom Frittata

Prep Time: 20 minutes

Ingredients:

2 eggs

1/4 cup chopped spinach

1/4 cup sliced mushrooms

1 tablespoon grated Parmesan cheese

Salt and pepper to taste

Instructions:

Preheat oven to 350°F (175°C).

In a bowl, beat eggs and season with salt and pepper.

Heat an oven-safe skillet over medium heat and lightly coat with cooking spray.

Add chopped spinach and sliced mushrooms to the skillet and sauté until softened.

Pour beaten eggs over the vegetables in the skillet.

Cook for 3-4 minutes until the edges begin to set.

Sprinkle grated Parmesan cheese over the frittata.

Transfer the skillet to the preheated oven and bake for 10-12 minutes until the frittata is set and golden brown.

Calories: 250

Lunch: Turkey and Avocado Wrap

Prep Time: 10 minutes

Ingredients:

2 oz sliced turkey breast

1 whole wheat tortilla

1/4 avocado, mashed

1/4 cup shredded lettuce

1 tablespoon salsa

Instructions:

Lay the tortilla flat and spread mashed avocado over it.

Layer sliced turkey breast, shredded lettuce, and salsa on top of the avocado.

Roll up the tortilla and serve.

Calories: 300

Dinner: Baked Cod with Lemon Garlic Butter Sauce

Prep Time: 25 minutes

Ingredients:

4 oz cod fillet

1 teaspoon olive oil

1/2 tablespoon lemon juice

1/2 teaspoon minced garlic

1/2 tablespoon chopped fresh parsley

Salt and pepper to taste

Instructions:

Preheat oven to 375°F (190°C).

Place cod fillet on a baking sheet lined with parchment paper.

Drizzle with olive oil and lemon juice. Season with minced garlic, chopped fresh parsley, salt, and pepper.

Bake for 12-15 minutes or until fish is opaque and flakes easily with a fork.

Calories: 300

Snack: Greek Yogurt with Almonds

Prep Time: 5 minutes

Ingredients:

1/2 cup plain Greek yogurt

1 tablespoon sliced almonds

Instructions:

Top Greek yogurt with sliced almonds.

Calories: 150

CONCLUSION

In concluding our journey through the pages of this cookbook, it is with utmost gratitude and hope that I extend my deepest appreciation to you, dear reader. Together, we have explored the intricacies of stage 3 kidney disease and delved into the realm of nourishing recipes designed to support and enhance kidney health.

As we reach the end of this culinary expedition, it is imperative to reflect on the profound impact that food can have on our well-being. Through careful consideration of ingredients, portion sizes, and cooking methods, we have crafted a collection of recipes that not only tantalize the taste buds but also nourish the body from within.

From hearty breakfasts to satisfying dinners, each dish has been thoughtfully curated to provide essential nutrients while minimizing the burden on compromised kidneys. By embracing wholesome ingredients and mindful eating habits, we can harness the power of food to promote healing, vitality, and overall wellness.

But our journey does not end here. As you embark on your own culinary adventures, I encourage you to continue exploring the vast array of flavors and ingredients available to you. Let this cookbook serve as a foundation upon which to build a lifetime of healthy eating habits and culinary creativity.

Remember, the path to wellness is not always linear, and setbacks may occur along the way. Yet, with determination, resilience, and the nourishing power of food by your side, you possess the tools needed to navigate the challenges that lie ahead.

As you turn the final page of this cookbook, may you carry with you a renewed sense of purpose and empowerment. May you savor each bite with gratitude and intention, knowing that you are nourishing not only your body but also your soul.

Thank you for entrusting me with your journey to kidney health. May your path be filled with abundance, vitality, and the joy of wholesome eating. Wishing you continued health and happiness on your culinary adventure.

With warmest regards,

LAURA B. COLLINS